CW01560551

ISBN 9798670355292

Please write to us with your experience on this program:

HealingEdition@gmail.com

This book is dedicated to all those who suffer from multiple sclerosis.

There is light at the end of the tunnel.

Contents

Introduction

Multiple sclerosis begins when myelin—the protective shell around a nerve—is damaged in the brain and spinal cord. The term *sclerosis* refers to the damaged areas of myelin.

Inflammation is responsible for damaging the brain's hematoencephalic barrier, breaking down proteins, and making the barrier porous (Letarte, 2019). This porosity allows inflammatory molecules to reach the brain and attack tissues, including myelin.

When the body is injured, inflammation occurs to facilitate healing or defend against a potential threat. Threats are usually in the form of viruses, bacteria, fungi, parasites, etc., and inflammation is essential to healing. During the healing process, white blood cells overcome bacteria and other cells, and they remove dead cells in the affected area. Acute inflammation usually disappears within a few days when these repairs are done.

But when inflammation becomes chronic, it no longer serves its healing purpose, which becomes a problem. Chronic inflammation is a low-grade reaction; there is no swelling (like when you are injured), but it damages human tissues, which leads to disease.

Modern medicine is highly successful in curing certain diseases, but not others. Modern medicine considers Multiple

Sclerosis to be an irreversible condition; there is no magic pill to cure the disease. With inflammatory and most chronic diseases, what is available is some degree of symptom relief with medication—but the effects tend to decrease over time; as the disease progresses, medication becomes less effective.

Inflammation becomes chronic when its causes persist. The body tries to rid itself of the problem repeatedly, without success. Toxins accumulate and trigger more inflammation. We will examine the different sources of inflammation and how to avoid the toxic build-up. So, to cure Multiple Sclerosis, you must eliminate the sources of toxins that trigger inflammation. Once the inflammation is gone, your myelin will be able to restore itself and the healing process will begin.

The study and diet explained in this book were followed by 46 patients. 13 patients experienced a complete remission, 20 patients a clear improvement and 8 patients a 50% improvement. Only 1 patient did not experience any improvement. These results are well above any placebo effect, prescribed medication, or medical treatment, as there is no complete remission with conventional medicine.

Chapter 1: The Agricultural Revolution and Multiple Sclerosis

The main source of disease in humans comes from food and water, our primary contacts with the external world. Foods are reduced from complex to simple chemicals by the digestive system for use by our cells. Carbohydrates and fats give us energy while proteins are the building blocks for repairing the body. When we ate whole and natural foods in their original forms—picked fresh in the wild—there was a healthy balance of carbohydrates, fiber, vitamins, minerals, proteins and water.

Our only source of energy comes from food, so it's the place to look for answers. The word "diet" means "way of life," in Greek. So, *to diet* is to change your way of life—to eat better. The Paleo diet movement offers the first clue to providing answers; our bodies were not designed to eat the foods we eat today. For millions of years, we were hunter-gatherers eating raw fruits, tubers and vegetables picked on the move, catching fish, and hunting animals for meat. Our bodies evolved with these foods and the digestive system adapted, producing the gastric enzymes needed to break down these molecules for optimal assimilation. The fruits and vegetables in this diet were high in fiber, which allowed quick bowel transit that avoided food putrefaction in the gut. The only milk product was consumed during breastfeeding in early childhood, but none was eaten later. We were eating low-fat proteins that made humans taller. There was little tooth decay or degenerative disease. Humans had high energy levels that allowed them to move across vast distances around the globe.

Though the Paleo diet is well adapted to the body, I would not necessarily recommend it because it is very limiting in food choices. It is possible to have more choices, but still respect the way the body functions. For example, rice is not allowed in the Paleo diet, but it is well tolerated by the digestive system, in contrast to wheat. And rice provides multiple food options including rice milk or bread, which can replace conventional cow milk or wheat bread.

The agricultural revolution

Eleven thousand years ago an agricultural revolution began, and it has defined what we are today—for better or worse. Humans realized that when the grains of plants like wheat scattered in the wind, they grew where they landed. People began to pick up these grains, not to eat them immediately but to plant them to produce more. This was a great idea because it provided a reliable and plentiful food supply. This was the first time humans had some control over the amount of food that might be available to them. Imagine being limited to the food you could pick up along the way, like fruits and vegetables, or animals you had to hunt to be able to eat.

Of course, fruits and vegetables were only available part of the year, weather permitting. And not being able to find enough animals to kill could mean death for the whole clan. Humans went from an uncertain food supply to planning how much they could grow. This change was a true revolution that brought great benefits: food in sufficient amounts that could be stored for when it was needed.

The consequences of this revolution

However, during this transition we abandoned the variety we had previously enjoyed. Humans began to eat fewer types of food and some rarely eaten before: grains, and milk products from domesticated animals—digestion of these new foods was less than optimal. Carbohydrate intake went up and protein intake went down, and the array of modern degenerative diseases began to appear. The fossils of our ancestors show this health decline: tooth decay, lower bone density, and anemia from iron deficiency became widespread. Humans consumed fewer vitamins and minerals with this new diet, so we became shorter and the infant mortality rate increased. Evidence suggests that early farmers who depended on one or two starchy crops to survive, like wheat or corn, developed vitamin-deficiency diseases such as beriberi or scurvy that had not been seen before.

Can your digestive system break down the foods you eat?

The body's enzymes were not designed to break down these new foods, the grains and milk products; they had developed specifically to digest the foods we had been eating for millions of years, namely fruits, vegetables and meat proteins (Kresser, 2013). If you think we should have adapted to grains and milk products by now, consider 10,000 years versus the four million years we ate our original diet. Ten thousand years is really the blink of an eye in the human evolutionary process. Consequently, foods no longer were being properly broken down, and larger molecules that the body could not absorb began accumulating.

The vital part that enzymes play

Enzymes are crucial for maintaining proper digestion and good health. They are proteins in the digestive system that accelerate the chemical reactions needed to break down food. A reaction that could take days or months without enzymes can happen in seconds with them. Very few enzymes are needed to transform millions of molecules so that the body can absorb nutrients. But enzymes are highly specialized—each only transforms one type of molecule, affecting only one type of reaction. If what we eat is designed for a specific enzyme, that enzyme will break down that food very efficiently. But when we started to eat new types of foods like grains or milk products, there were no enzymes available to break them down—and that is where our problems began. For example, people with lactose intolerance can't digest the sugar in milk, but a lactase enzyme supplement can be taken to digest milk sugar. Among the 2,700 enzymes that have been identified to date, some partially break down these new foods, but only up to a point (Lipski, 2013).

How to help your enzymes

You can help your enzymes function properly by taking minerals like magnesium, calcium, iron or zinc (themedicalbiochemistrypage.org, s.d.).

If you have difficulty with digestion, you can also take vegetable enzyme supplements that can be bought at any store selling natural products. But, in the end, if there is no enzyme that breaks down a specific food, the problem remains. Enzymes are the key to understanding why the modern diet is creating health problems. However, we can reverse health problems like multiple sclerosis if we go back to eating foods the digestive system was designed for.

Eating grains as gatherers

In our hunter-gatherer prehistoric past, we ate grains from wild wheat, oats, barley or rye that were found along the way. But the supply was not constant, and quantities were restricted because there were no cultivated fields, as there are today—the plants were scattered. These grains were hard to chew in their original state so not much could be eaten at one time. Occasionally, even when these smaller amounts were eaten, the body had a hard time with digestion. But the amount of undigested larger molecules was small, and the body had time to recover, until the next time the same food was eaten.

The immune reaction to food that triggers inflammation

However, when large amounts of food that can't be broken down properly are eaten, and when this is done again and again over a long period of time, a problem occurs. First, the digestive system does not recognize these undigested larger molecules and reacts to them as a threat. The immune system attacks these molecules to try to get rid of them, which triggers inflammation (Hyman M. , 2009). This is not acute inflammation, as would occur with an injury; it is a low-grade inflammation reaction that worsens over time. Because these grains and milk products became the new staple foods, the body continued to react to them. When the body can no longer rid itself of this toxin buildup, chronic inflammation begins. These changes occurred too quickly to allow the human body to evolve; our physiology has remained the same since our prehistoric past.

Solving enzyme deficiency

Today, many suffer from digestive enzyme deficiencies and they are unable to digest what others can. This problem tends to worsen as we get older. At age 50, there is about 50% enzyme deficiency: at age 60, 60%, and so on (Lipski, 2013). Therefore, if you have a health problem like multiple sclerosis, it is helpful to take digestive enzymes to make sure your food is properly broken down, so it doesn't end up triggering inflammation in your system. We need the lipase enzyme to break down fats, protease for proteins, and amylase for carbohydrates.

The calorie source change

Another way to measure this dramatic change is by looking at various calorie sources (EATON):

Before 10000 BC, humans consumed:

33% proteins

22% fats

45% carbohydrates, rich in fiber (raw whole foods)

No white sugar or lactose from milk

After the agricultural revolution, humans consumed:

11% proteins

37% fats

52% total carbohydrates, converted and low in fiber

27% white sugar and 5% lactose

Now, our intake of proteins, which are the building blocks of the body, is drastically reduced but the meat we eat is much fatter than what was consumed when we were hunter-gatherers. Our fat consumption has nearly doubled, and our sugar consumption went from virtually nothing to one quarter of our calorie intake. This has created today's obesity and diabetes crises, although they are just the most visible aspects of the damage being done.

The problem with wheat

Wheat and barley became the main part of the typical diet along with the milk products resulting from the domestication of cows and goats. Imagine that you filled your car's diesel engine with regular unleaded gas; the engine would slowly break down because it is not meant to run on this type of fuel, even though it is made for car engines. The same goes for the human body—even if we can eat something, it does not mean that the body has the enzymes needed to break it down. Grains and milk products are broken down to a certain extent, but not enough for the body to function properly in the long run. Those toxic bigger molecules—as with unleaded gas in a diesel engine—accumulate in the digestive system and create inflammation and disease over the years (Permutter, 2015).

Food intolerance

The food we eat was not created to be eaten by us. The plants and other products we eat are alien to the human body and some of us will have allergic reactions to them, which means the body rejects an external element that is deemed to be dangerous.

But even without an allergic reaction, many of us will have some reaction or degree of intolerance to certain foods that can make one feel tired, depressed or irritable. These symptoms can be felt a few hours or days after eating. Even if you don't have a severe allergic reaction to a food, your body can react in a more subtly intolerant way that can lead to inflammation (Brostoff, 2000).

We are not designed to eat the new foods in our diet, namely wheat and milk, because we are not capable of digesting them properly. But we now continually eat these foods in large amounts, to a point where the digestive system cannot eliminate toxins fast enough to maintain its balance. Cytokines from the immune system attack these toxins and inflammation occurs. Because we keep ingesting more toxins in the foods we eat, inflammation becomes chronic, as it does for multiple sclerosis patients. We will explore different foods that can trigger inflammation in the digestive system and that should be avoided.

Chapter 2: The Industrial Revolution: A Disaster for Multiple sclerosis

The agricultural revolution—the first evolution in the way humans ate—was damaging enough to health as the result of all the new foods the body could not digest properly. However, the second revolution was even worse; it began around 1850 with the introduction of industrialization. New machines and processes dramatically changed humans' relation to food. Prior to industrialization, we prepared and cooked the wholesome foods we ate. Mass production introduced altered foods, transformed from their original state. In the last few decades, low quality, over the counter, ready-cooked meals and fast foods flooded the market, taking the place of home-made, wholesome meals.

Also, all of these cheap and unhealthy products could be moved over vast distances using more efficient transportation when railroads were introduced. During the early 1900s, most of the population in North America and Europe had access to this industrialized food, which was mainly produced from wheat, corn and potatoes. As cars became affordable, humans became more sedentary in general, walked much less, drove more, and burned fewer calories. This happened while our calorie intake from processed foods increased—a recipe for disaster because the number of calories we now eat is greater than the amount we burn, which has become the obesity crisis we are currently experiencing.

White flour

Around 1850, the flour industry began separating the different components of grains: bran (or fiber) and germs were removed to produce white flour, which is essentially pure starch. This doesn't seem important, but it is. This is the first time in human history that starch was eaten without the fiber and proteins. Half a cup of whole wheat flour contains about 6.4 grams of fiber while the same amount of white flour contains about 1.3 grams (Tremblay, 2018). Therefore, there is about 5 times more fiber in whole-grain flour. Eating whole-grain flour that contains fiber slows down the digestion of carbohydrates, avoiding a rapid rise in blood sugar. Fiber is a brake pedal in the absorption of carbohydrates.

The absence of fiber allows us to eat faster, and the sweeter taste of white flour makes us eat more; we don't feel as satiated as when we eat whole foods. A large intake of carbohydrates creates a rapid increase in blood sugar such that our bodies had never before experienced. These days, this is not a once-in-a-while occurrence—now it's all day every day, which wears down our ability to manage constant blood sugar spikes.

The Glycemic Index (GI) measures how fast the body absorbs carbohydrates. Bread made with whole flour has a GI of 50; bread made with white flour has a GI of 70 (Tremblay, 2018).

This means that the speed of absorption of white flour is 40% faster, which is dramatic for one's body because blood sugar spikes and then crashes soon after, causing you to become irritable, in a rage for more sugar that causes another blood sugar spike—and the cycle endlessly repeats itself.

Eating whole-grain flour makes you feel satisfied much longer because you don't have that blood sugar spike and crash. However, white flour is just one of many products popular today that causes blood sugar spikes. A similar analysis can be done for products containing sugar, like sweet beverages or alcohol. These have all caused the diabetes crisis that began in Western countries; the disease was almost non-existent before industrialization.

Another problem with industrialized foods is that the mechanical processes that are used tend to strip out the vitamins, minerals and nutrients found in whole foods, which we need to function efficiently. For example, whole wheat flour contains 3 milligrams of niacin, an essential vitamin for the body. White flour only has 0.8 milligrams of niacin—three times less (Tremblay, 2018). The same can be said for other vitamins and minerals, so we end up eating empty calories with little beneficial content in comparison with what we should have.

Sugar and inflammation

Before industrialization, sugar intake was from fruits that had fiber, which slowed down the absorption process. But with industrialization, cane or beet sugar was introduced that is absorbed quickly into our blood stream. Then fruit juices and sodas were introduced; they contain around 8 teaspoons of liquid sugar that is absorbed at lightning speed for a 12-oz portion (Bowers, 2020). A large format iced cappuccino has an astounding 18 tablespoons of sugar! Sugar consumption in the UK went from less than 5 pounds in 1700 to more than 100 pounds in 2000 (Yudkin, 2012). The body is not designed to deal with such high amounts of sugar that are absorbed so quickly, and there are serious repercussions for this.

Consuming high amounts of sugar leads to obesity and diabetes, which has reached epidemic proportions around the world, but it is also a problem if you suffer from multiple sclerosis. The link is simple: too much sugar will ferment in the gut and lead to a yeast overgrowth, Candida albicans (Martin, 2000). This yeast, when it takes over the normal flora of the gut, attacks the gut lining and eventually makes it permeable. A permeable or leaky gut allows bigger food molecules into the internal system, but the body does not recognize them as safe, so they are attacked by the immune system via cytokines and inflammation.

The effects of sugar spikes

The only sugar we should eat should come from whole, raw fruits because they are balanced in their water, fiber and sugar content; and, the fiber slows down the absorption process. Typically, your blood sugar will not have a big spike when you eat fruit, unlike when you drink soda. Liquid sugar, which is in all sweet drinks, is the number one cause of wild swings in blood sugar—it goes up dramatically and then crashes down, making you feel irritated or depressed, depending on the individual. You then feel compelled to eat more sugar to make you feel high again, until the next sugar crash.

Sugar: A drug?

The same process happens with drug users—they always need their next high. Refined sugar is not whole-fruit sugar; it is a drug that stimulates the regions of the brain associated with pleasure, the same regions affected in drug addicts, and our serotonin level spikes dramatically (Appleton, 2009). That's why it's so hard to resist refined sugar. Any sugar that is quickly absorbed, whether from a dessert or a sweet drink, will have the same effect on one's state of mind. When there's a sugar crash, you tend to eat more and a lot faster, which makes you gain weight. Will power goes out the window with such a strong stimulant, and your rational side is unable to resist the rush a body experiences during a sugar spike.

Hidden sugars

So many hidden sugars are now added to foods, but most people don't even suspect them. Most of our processed foods contain added sugar that contributes to our sugar addiction. Soups, crackers, yogurts, tomato sauces and all the other processed staple products we eat have added sugar for the express purpose of making them irresistible to our taste buds. Commercial ketchup or yogurt, for example, contain about one third sugar; barbecue sauce is more than half sugar. This added sugar causes us to crave it more, adding more profit to the bottom line of the major food corporations. Half the sugar we consume comes from added sugar.

Here is a list of products containing sugar that we don't necessarily suspect:

Breads

Muffins

Bagels

Tomato sauce

Mayonnaise

Ketchup (25% sugar minimum)

Relish

Soups, even those that don't taste sweet

Pickles

Corn syrup, etc.

Recognizing different kinds of sugar

To identify sugar content, we must read food labels. But this is tricky because sugar hides behind many names in an ingredient list. *Sugar* can be white cane sugar, beet sugar or molasses—these are the conventional ones. But fructose, glucose, agave syrup, honey, corn syrup, maple syrup and others are also sugars.

A major problem: High fructose corn syrup

The most recent addition to the list is high fructose corn syrup. It appeared in the 1980s as a consequence of industrialization, flooding the market because it is less expensive (half the price of sugar) and sweeter than conventional sugar. It is found in sodas, among other things. This was a bonus for industrial producers because it costs less and is even more addictive than sugar. High fructose syrup is composed of 55% fructose and 45% glucose versus 50% fructose and 50% glucose for white sugar (Mawer, 2019). This seems like a small difference, but it has a big impact on the body's ability to resist these products and on overall health. The main problem with high fructose corn syrup is that it doesn't trigger the feeling of satiety that tells us it's time to stop eating (Kleiner, 2003). As a result, we end up eating more high-calorie products than we should.

High fructose corn syrup makes us fat

After the introduction of high fructose corn syrup, there was an explosion of obesity and diabetes in Western societies in the 1980s. Americans eat on average 37 lbs of HFCS per year (Statista, 2018). We gained weight because a percentage of high fructose corn syrup consumed is converted directly into fat by the liver. You can gain up to 3 times more weight by consuming HFCS than by consuming fruit sugar (Group, 2015). Diet products on the market contain less fat, but the fat is often replaced by high fructose corn syrup, which turns into fat anyway—so it's a losing battle. In the long run, this fat—the worst kind—accumulates in one's organs, makes blood sugar levels go up, and leads to type 2 diabetes, but also to a significant increase of inflammation (MAWER, 2019) in the case of Multiple Sclerosis.

High fructose corn syrup toxins

High fructose corn syrup contains up to 10 times more advanced glycation end products (AGE) than regular sugar (Gugliucci, 2017). These are the toxins that lead to inflammation. And high fructose corn syrup is in most of the processed foods we buy at the supermarket. It is found in breads, soups, cookies, condiments, etc. Just read the labels—it's everywhere! Therefore, it's important to avoid processed foods and to buy whole foods that you cook yourself. If you don't always have time to cook, buying organic processed foods is a better choice because these usually contain natural and simple ingredients—but you still have to read the label to make sure. All of these small steps will help reduce your suffering.

High fructose corn syrup is only metabolized by the liver, the same as alcohol. You can develop hepatic liver problems due to chronic high fructose consumption as well as other alcohol-related problems because the liver processes them both in the same way (Group, 2015).

Stick to whole fruits

Metabolizing fructose from fruit is easy for the liver since fruit has little sugar compared to a fruit drink or soda, and digestion is slowed down by the fiber. As a result, the fruit will be well absorbed, and you also get the fiber, vitamins and minerals your body needs. Favor organic fruits, free of pesticides or herbicides like glyphosate, to decrease your chances of developing a cancer later in life. If organically grown produce is just too expensive for your budget, choose fruits than can be easily washed with a brush or peeled to remove most residual chemicals. Avoid fruit that can't be brushed easily, like grapes; washing grapes in water is just not enough because pesticides will remain.

It is best to cut out all fruit drinks, not just sodas. Both are concentrated sources of fructose with no fiber to slow down the absorption, even if their ingredients are from natural sources. Any fructose, and sugar in general, should be eaten with plenty of fiber. Also, energy drinks contain multiple stimulant chemicals that can be harmful to your gut and inflamed joints, so they should be completely avoided, too.

When you drink a glass of orange juice, you drink about 5 or 6 orange at once. All this sugar rapidly enters the blood stream, causing a sugar crash. You would not eat 6 oranges at once in real life. Clearly, there is a big difference between the fruit and the drinks concerning the amounts ingested and the speeds of absorption.

Avoid the fruit rolls that many parents add to their kids' lunch. These have a very high sugar concentration and lack the fiber and water content of a fruit. Fruit rolls are as bad as eating a chocolate bar—instead, give children a real fruit. Kids have sugar crashes and get diabetes, too, and it's very hard to learn at school when blood sugar is too low, making concentration difficult. Many kids who are considered to have attention deficit suffer from sugar crashes throughout the day, but the real problem is the result of the liquid sugar they consume.

When eating real fruit, its taste is not strong enough to cause dependence, always wanting more—like a chocolate bar, for example. Let's say it like it is—all commercial candies are powerful drugs and it's almost impossible to stop eating them when we should. We eat too much because we simply can't stop ourselves, and we constantly need our drug. Concentrated sugar in candies is a legal drug. Nevertheless, it's a drug, and we should treat it as such if we want to break the cycle of eating it. At first, it will be very hard not to reach for sweets because we crave our drug rush. But if you can manage a few days without sweets, you will feel better and you won't need them as much anymore, as long as you don't backslide. In my experience, within three or four days you won't crave them as much. Eating enough fruit should help break the habit and your dependence on refined sugars.

Your body needs glucose

Conventional sugar is not good for anyone, but high fructose corn syrup is even worse. We don't need *any* refined sugar in our food. It is always best to stick to glucose from complex carbohydrates like bread or gluten-free pasta (not made with wheat and gluten grains, as will be explained). All cells in the body use glucose; glucose is what is needed to make us feel full. If you feel full but are still hungry, this is because glucose takes about 20 minutes to be absorbed by the body. So just stop eating when full and the hunger will disappear. Glucose, especially when it comes from whole foods that contain fiber, will not cause a blood sugar spike—as refined sugar does—so you will not experience a sugar crash and then need to binge eat. Remember that less sugar fermenting in your gut will lead to less inflammation.

Ending sugar addiction

The only way to end a sugar addiction is to ban liquid sugars from one's diet because they are the worst offenders. Liquid sugar is a quick and easy way to absorb large amounts of sugar, although too fast for your body to handle properly. This is exactly why authorities in many countries have approved additional taxes on sodas, which has significantly reduced consumption of these disaster drinks in those countries. Mexico applied an additional tax to reduce the diabetes epidemic in that country, which helped reduce the sugar consumption.

Processed foods.

Another way to end sugar addiction is to eat the lowest-possible amount of refined products—or ban them altogether from your grocery cart. The added sugars in our foods make us overeat because they are scientifically engineered to be irresistible. The food industry adds the maximum amount of sugar and salt possible in each food so that we can't resist their products. These added sugars also increase one's taste for sugar, and we tend to want more when we start having some.

Going back to eating wholesome foods with simple ingredients allows one's metabolism to slowly get back to normal, to the point where you won't be compelled by the taste of food to always eat more than you need. Your blood sugar will stabilize, the roller coaster effect will stop, you won't experience sugar crashes anymore, and you will just feel good again. It takes about three days for sugar cravings to end when I stop. But I eat very little sugar and it can take longer if you are strongly addicted. Organic products tend to use less sugar in general but read labels because many of them still do contain high amounts, even if they are natural sugars.

Chapter 3: Problem Foods?

Grains and wheat

Before the development of agriculture, small amounts of grain and wheat were consumed in comparison with today's consumption. They were consumed raw and whole including their cellulose fiber. We now eat mainly processed grains, which means we eat a lot more starch but up to 90% less fiber, and fewer proteins, vitamins and minerals. We also cook it, which changes the structure of the grain.

Over the centuries, as agriculture was being perfected, our ancestors didn't just plant grains, they selected the biggest grains to plant the next season. Bigger grains contain certain genetic mutations that make them bigger. Over time, the proteins in these grains became different from those in the original field plants that existed during the hunter-gatherer period. The ancestral grains of wheat had seven chromosomes, but the hard wheat now used to make pasta has 14 chromosomes and soft wheat used to make bread now has 21 chromosomes (Seignalet, 2012). This is a major transformation considering that our enzymes have not had time to adjust to these changes. Similar modifications also occurred with other grains. Kamut, which is advertised as an ancestral wheat, also contains 14 chromosomes instead of seven, so it must also be avoided. Barley, rye, spelt and oats each have seven chromosomes but contain gluten, avoided because it irritates the gut and triggers inflammation.

Are wheat and gluten really that bad?

Many multiple sclerosis sufferers find that their symptoms ease after a few months when they cut wheat and other gluten grains, but that their symptoms reappears if they start to eat them again. After fasting a few days, many multiple sclerosis sufferers feel that their symptoms go away. One study shows that 54% of arthritis sufferers say their symptoms return after the reintroduction of wheat (Darlington, 1986) So yes, wheat and other glutens grains are *that* bad for inflammation.

Corn

Corn is another example of these mutations. Originally, a corn cob was small, measuring about 1 inch. Selection of the best and biggest kernels each year led to the six- to nine-inch-long corn cobs we have today. These have little in common with their ancestors because major mutations occurred during this selection process. Corn is another example of a new food that is now consumed in large quantities that the body was not designed to digest properly. Therefore, any products related to corn should be avoided including corn flour, corn flakes, popped corn, chips containing corn as an ingredient, etc. If this is hard to believe, think of regular unleaded gas when it's put into a diesel engine—it will ruin the motor, even though both types of gas are made to run motors. Corn and gluten can ruin your gut balance, creating inflammation and autoimmune diseases. After fasting a few days, many multiple sclerosis sufferers feel that their symptoms go away. 56% of arthritis sufferers say their symptoms return after the reintroduction of corn (Darlington, 1986), a percentage higher than with wheat.

Rice

Rice is different; when it is manipulated, it tends to return to its original state over time and its structure has not changed since the agricultural age began (Seignalet, 2012). It's also a food that, in general, does not cause allergic reactions or intolerance, as gluten does.

Watch for arsenic in rice

Rice is now cultivated everywhere on the planet but try to avoid North American rice. In the areas where it's cultivated in North America, the soil has a high level of arsenic that could make you sick overtime, especially if consumed as brown rice.

Rice from China can also be a problem because many of the rivers that irrigate the rice fields are contaminated with heavy metals like cadmium as a result of industrial pollution. It's best to geographically vary the sources of your rice to avoid long-term issues. Now, many rice varieties come from different parts of India or Pakistan.

Even organic rice can be contaminated with arsenic. This is because the contamination is present in the soil—the arsenic does not come from added pesticides. It's best to be aware that higher levels of arsenic than those currently allowed have been found in baby foods made with North American brown rice. Any brown rice product made in North America will most likely be made from North American rice and should be consumed with moderation. For example, the rice milk I use is made in Italy, with locally grown Italian rice—I geographically vary the rice products I buy.

Milk products

For millions of years, our human ancestors only drank mother's milk as babies, but not a drop after. This is the only milk our species was designed to consume, and only at a young age.

Suddenly, 10,000 years ago, we started drinking milk as adults and eating all sorts of milk-derived substances (yogurt, cheese, butter, etc.) in large quantities. These milk products did not come from our own species—they came from other species: cows, goats, sheep. Prior to this, humans as well as all other animals on earth never drank milk as an adult, and never from another species.

Consuming cow milk as adults is a new habit, although it seems normal now because it's widespread. However, it is anything but normal—a good example of how human perception can affect reality if enough people do it. There are significant differences between a human mother's milk and cow milk. Cow milk contains 2 times more protein, but not the same types of protein as in human milk and they are not adapted to human digestion and physiology (D'souza, 2015). This abnormal habit is causing big problems in human health. We were never able or meant to digest cow milk and there are consequences when we do.

The milk-product industry has even convinced us through marketing that the calcium in cow milk is essential for our bones. In truth, cow milk is poorly absorbed by the body. Even worse, cow milk products deplete the calcium in the body. This happens because protein-rich cow milk lowers the body's pH level, making it acidic, so that calcium is taken from the bones to balance the pH level—the perfect example of how good marketing can be bad for your health.

Many arthritis sufferers experience a remission when they stop consuming milk products, and the reintroduction of milk products is followed by the return of arthritic symptoms (Darlington, 1986). So yes, milk is also *that bad* for inflammation.

Eggs

Many people are allergic to eggs, which shows that the body can severely react to them, so it's best to avoid them. Before the agricultural revolution, eggs were rarely eaten—only when one was found along the way. Our enzymes are not designed for digesting eggs. We used to eat them in very small quantities but today we consume large amounts, which trigger inflammation reactions.

When I stopped eating eggs for one month, I felt my energy level go up significantly, and when I started eating them again, I became tired and depressed—so I stopped eating eggs entirely. Even if you are not allergic to eggs, when you eat them you can still have an intolerance with an array of symptoms and inflammation.

Soy

Soy is another example of a product rarely consumed before the agricultural age and that has become a large portion of the food eaten, especially by vegetarians who use it as a meat substitute. Again, the body is not designed to digest this new food, therefore many people are allergic or have an intolerance to it.

Another problem is that farmers in many countries use glyphosate, an herbicide, to kill soy plants, lentils and peas before harvesting them, which saves money by speeding up the drying process. High trace amounts of glyphosate are on these plants because spraying is done just before harvesting. In 2015, the World Health Organization (through its International Agency for Research on Cancer) and the European Food Safety Authority labeled glyphosate a probable cancer agent for humans. But to this day, glyphosate is still being used extensively in conventional agriculture. Glyphosate, a very harmful chemical, can also trigger inflammation.

Glyphosate limits in food supplies can vary greatly from one country to the next. In the Europe Union, the maximum level in many countries is 0.1 ppm (parts per million), but in Canada and the U.S. it's around 10 ppm, or 100 times higher. Don't count on the maximum level allowed in North America to shield you from the devastating problems glyphosate can cause—North American limits are way too high and out of control. The limits have increased over time because of pressures from the chemical industry. This is an example of regulators listening to the chemical industry instead of using common sense and reserve when dealing with a potential cancer agent.

The practice of drying crops with glyphosate is widespread in North America for grains like wheat and oats. Only organic foods can shield you from harmful glyphosate exposure because this herbicide is forbidden for use in organic agriculture.

Potatoes

Potatoes are usually well tolerated by most people when they are boiled. When they are fried and become our famous French fries or chips, the frying process produces acrylamides, which are very toxic molecules that are highly suspected of causing cancer (Cancer.org, 2019) and inflammation.

If you like the crunchy taste of chips, try the low-fat baked versions—or puffed rice cakes—that are much better for avoiding inflammation.

Quinoa, Millet, buckwheat

These grains don't have gluten, but are new to humanity in most regions, so like wheat your system doesn't have the enzymes to digest them. So, by eating them you run the risk of having your immune system react to them with inflammation. If you eat them, make sure it's not on a regular basis.

Legumes

Legumes were part of the hunter-gatherer's diet, but not in quantity. They can be used occasionally, just not on a regular basis. Sprouted legumes, which are live food, are best because vitamins and nutrients are at their peak.

Vegetables

Vegetables like broccoli, cabbage and collard greens have been shown to reduce the risk of many cancers. All vegetables are alkaline and contain phytochemicals, which reduce inflammation. Raw vegetables are the preferred choice—they retain all their vitamins and minerals. But if you don't like raw vegetables, lightly stir-fry them with gluten-free soy sauce for added flavor. The darker the color of fruits or vegetables, the more phytochemicals they contain.

Inflammation-fighting vegetables

Carrots, broccoli, cabbage, bok choy, cauliflower, kale, Brussels sprouts, green lettuce, spinach, collards, beans, sweet potatoes, red or green peppers, etc.

Inflammation-fighting fruits

Grapefruit, lime, lemon, orange, blackberries, blueberries, raspberries, strawberries, mango, cantaloupe, pumpkin, kiwi, etc.

Other vegetables and fruits will help reduce inflammation as well. Try to eat as much of them as possible every day to boost your inflammation-fighting abilities with phytochemicals. But they must be organic or you will end up eating a lot of residual herbicides/pesticides that can worsen your inflammation.

Increase your vegetable consumption

Sandwiches

To increase your vegetable intake, you can reduce the amount of meat in your next sandwich and increase the greens, tomatoes and other veggies. Why not add slices of green, red or orange peppers, olives, and spread avocado instead of using mayonnaise (to avoid eggs). Use rice or tapioca breads, rice pitas and other gluten-free choices.

Green salads

Add beans, seeds and multiple fruits or organic dried fruits (without preservation additives) to add color and taste; blend with flaked salmon to get omega 3 oils. Use flaxseed oil instead of inflammation-triggering heated vegetable oil; flaxseed contains omega 6, which can reduce inflammation.

Snacks

Instead of eating high-sugar cereal bars try baby carrots and any other raw vegetables, mixed with fresh-cut fruits or organic dried fruits and nuts. Nuts will slow down absorption of the dried fruit. Or try a fruit shake drink mixed with nut or bean protein powder (to reduce the speed of sugar absorption). Why not even have a salad with nuts or dried salmon in the afternoon instead of high-sugar snacks. These c

changes will have a huge impact on your multiple sclerosis.

Fish

Adding fish to your diet a few times a week will help reduce inflammation because it contains omega-3 fatty acids that are anti-inflammatory fats. Omega-3 suppresses the production of inflammation (CALDER, 2017). For example, the Innu eat a large amount of fish and had virtually no Western diseases (heart disease, cancers, diabetes), until they recently began to adopt a Western diet. Now there has been an explosion in diabetes and other diseases previously unknown in that population.

Adding omega 3

Omega-3 from fish lowers inflammation. The best fish for adding omega-3 to your diet are salmon, herring, trout, sardines and tuna. But limit tuna to once or twice per week since it contains higher levels of mercury. The goal is to consume fish three times per week.

Another way to consume omega-3 oils is to add fish oil or a tablespoon of flaxseed oil to salads as a supplement to your regular routine. Fish oil has been shown to reduce inflammation. If you don't like the taste of fish oil, you can get it in capsule form, to be taken with water or food to avoid the taste. To have an anti-inflammatory effect, the minimum amount is 500 milligrams per day (Mobbs, 2020).

Chapter 4: Other Sources of Inflammation

Salt

The body needs salt, but we eat way too much of it. Food manufacturers know that adding salt is a cheap way to instantly add taste—but most of all, it makes many foods addictive. Salt can be found in cheese, chips or deli meat, but it's also in every staple processed food we eat like bread, soup, spaghetti sauce, dressing, cereal, cookies, packaged and canned food, etc. On average, we each eat 3.4 g of salt per day but should not consume more than 2.3 g (Heart.org, 2020), which is approximately 50% more than is advised. This creates excess acid in the digestive system that can leads to inflammation.

Potassium is a substitute that can help reduce your salt intake, but it will alter the taste of your food if you use too much. Just a little adds a nice flavor. Reducing the salt in one's diet is most important, and this can be done slowly.

If you reduce your salt intake slowly, it has been shown that you will become used to the new amount of salt in your food and it will be as tasty as it had been. Since 2003, Great Britain has forced food manufacturers to reduce the amount of salt in processed food by 30%. Now, when the English travel to other countries, they are shocked by how salty the food is— they have become used to much less salt in the processed foods they eat. This is good news because much less salt is needed to feel satisfied.

Coffee

Coffee can be a problem. Coffee plants produce coffee beans to poison and kill the bugs that try to eat it. Humans like the stimulating effect they get from coffee; but it stands to reason that if it's an insecticide for bugs, it might not have a great effect on your gut—especially if it's already irritated by the other inflammatory foods you eat. People who stop drinking coffee are also surprised by how much better they sleep.

If you are addicted to coffee, slowly reduce your intake and then try a three-month break. If you see no change, you can reintroduce it into your diet to see what happens. But you also would have to avoid adding milk or cream to your coffee because we have already identified them as problem foods, and even a tiny amount can make your system react and your joints hurt. Instead, you could choose to add rice milk as a replacement for the inflammatory cow milk. There are also rice cream replacements available in natural food stores.

Staying awake at work without coffee

Since coffee is often used for staying awake during a long workday, many can't see how they could function without it while at work. At work, a good way to replace the coffee habit is to develop the healthy habit of walking up and down a stairway. Taking a few minutes to go up and down stairs will get you fully awake and energized for the next hour or two. If you do this exercise a few times a day, you will not only be awake but will be in much better shape, too. Instead of being exhausted after work and only able to watch television, you will be able to do different activities after the evening meal—maybe take up a sport like badminton or do yoga, which will help you be more focused and relaxed in your daily routine. All this exercise will help your bowel movement, decreasing food putrefaction in your gut and the toxins it produces. These are the benefits you'll experience when you use a better approach to staying awake at work—exercising instead of drinking coffee.

Tea

Tea is a much safer choice for your gut because it is not irritating like coffee and it contains polyphenols and antioxidants that can help reduce inflammation. For example, drinking green tea can reduce your risk of stomach cancer by 30% (Meggs, 2004)

The problem with tea is that many people feel they're drinking hot water because of the lack of taste. This is often the case when you buy a mass-produced commercial brand at the supermarket. But if you take time to explore higher quality natural brands, you will find many varieties of exotic blends to try and you will likely find one you enjoy, maybe one with dried berries. It won't be sweet like fruit juice—it's a more subtle taste you can learn to enjoy once your body is not drugged by the strong taste of sugar.

Medications

Prescription medication taken over an extended period can also become an issue. These chemicals can have side effects anywhere in the body and among them is inflammation. I am not advising that you stop taking life-saving medication, but sometimes pills are taken for small issues that could be dealt with differently.

This includes, of course, the non-prescription, over-the-counter medications used to ease symptoms but that may not be essential; they, too, contain chemicals or active ingredients that can cause inflammation. You may not know until you stop taking something whether or not it's affecting your inflammation. And just because the government tolerates the over-the-counter sale of a pill does not mean that it cannot be harmful to you. Your system can be more sensitive to a chemical than the general population's experience. Even if most people can tolerate a certain chemical, it doesn't mean that you won't have a reaction to it and that it won't cause damage if taken over an extended period.

Antacid

An example of a medication that is used in excess and that the body doesn't need is antacids for heartburn. These acid-blocking prescription medications, like Nexium or Pantozol, or the over-the-counter brands like Zantac or Prilosec, are among the top-selling drugs. These drugs ease discomfort in the short term but create a much bigger problem if taken long term. A high acid level in the stomach is essential for the absorption of nutrients such as calcium, magnesium and zinc, which are all indispensable for good health.

Stomach acid is also essential for protection against bacteria, fungi or parasites because these are mostly destroyed by stomach acid (Smith, 2003). Low stomach acid can lead to small intestinal bacterial overgrowth (SIBO). Bacteria that are not destroyed by stomach acid produce toxins affecting different functions in the body (even brain functions, like brain fog and depression) and creating inflammation. For the body to function properly, the stomach needs more acid rather than less.

Stomach acid blockers often are used to allow us to eat more of the foods we shouldn't eat, like pizza, when the body reacts to the excess with acid reflux. Stomach acid is not the problem—abusing the wrong foods is—pushing acid into the wrong place: the esophagus. If we stop eating fast food, we won't need the acid blockers that harm us by weakening the immune system and diminishing resistance to foreign invaders.

Low stomach acid can lead to indigestion, so you really don't want low stomach acid. Taking antacid becomes a vicious cycle: You might have indigestion because your stomach acid is too low, but you think your stomach acid is too high, so you take more antacid, which only makes your digestive problems worse.

Alternatives to antacids

Instead of an antacid, use a natural betaine hydrochloride (HCL) supplement with pepsin that helps digest meals by adding acid, which breaks down food molecules; more rather than less stomach acid is needed to digest properly (Wright, 2019).

You can also use certain plant enzymes to aide in better digestion. These enzymes are efficient at breaking down and assimilating food molecules. Look for enzymes containing bromelain, papain, pancreatin and protease, which are good for hard-to-digest proteins, and lipase for breaking down fats. Cellulase can break down hard-to-digest fiber and lactase can help with milk sugar. Lowering the stress level in your life will also help your body produce more protective stomach acid.

Natural supplements

Just because a product is natural doesn't mean *you* can tolerate it—even if most people can. Supplements contain all sorts of active ingredients that can have an effect. And even though a product is natural, it doesn't mean that it's better than a synthetic medication. Very harmful and poisonous substances can be found in nature. For example, opium is natural and it's not good for you. Natural supplements are also tricky because people sometimes take them for an extended period. They might be fine for a short period of time but, in the long run, they can accumulate in your system and trigger an inflammatory response. Again, even though the government allows the sale of a product, it can still produce low-grade inflammation. It's best to consider any natural supplement as a potential problem, and to consider stopping its use to see if your condition improves.

Many natural supplements don't provide the effects the manufacturer claims they will produce. Studies (if any) that demonstrate effectiveness often are done by the manufacturer and are skewed to show positive results. Even *independent* studies can be a problem because some manufacturers provide funding, which can influence results. The sugar industry, for example, may fund studies that claim sugar is not harmful to your health. They can then use these studies to attack rigorous studies. So always be cautious when reading the results of a study because it might be biased and funded by the industry.

Genetic predisposition

Some individuals have a genetic predisposition, defined as an increased likelihood of developing a disease. In these cases, an excess of toxins in the system can result in developing the diseases that usually affect the person's close family. Toxin surplus will result in Crohn's disease or multiple sclerosis if that particular disease is prevalent in a family's genetic history.

Genetic predisposition alone won't trigger a disease. However, combined with another factor (called a cofactor) such as the accumulation of toxins from the foods eaten, diseases can be triggered. By eliminating problematic foods and the toxins they generate, the symptoms and progression of disease will disappear. It's important to note that these improvements will last if a regime of toxin avoidance is followed, but they will reappear if old habits recur. Healing will be the result of a long-term lifestyle change.

Food additives

Additives have multiple uses in the food industry. They can be used as colorants or preservatives, but they are ultimately chemicals added to food that can trigger reactions from the immune system. They should all be avoided because you don't know which ones can trigger a reaction in your body.

When you don't recognize an ingredient on a label, it's generally not real food and it's best to avoid it. Nothing should be ignored, especially during the initial period of additive avoidance as you don't know which chemical can affect you. The best way to eat without chemical additives is to eat organically grown foods. This type of agriculture not only avoids herbicides and GMOs but aims to avoid chemical additives.

For optimal results, all industrialized or processed products should be avoided. Food should only have one ingredient, or very few. If a food has more, make sure they are all wholesome ingredients that exist in the real world and are not created artificially.

Any chemical added to your food is a potential problem for your health and can lead to inflammation. Even if a chemical is permitted by law, that doesn't mean it's good for you. Many reported side effects such as migraines, rashes, asthma, etc., are traced to food additives.

The most common additives are aspartame (artificial sweetener), monosodium glutamate (adds flavor), nitrites (antibacterial in processed meats), and sulphites (antibacterial added to wine and many bottled liquids like fruit juices or colas, even if not labeled as such). Manufacturers even add antibacterial agents to dried fruits.

There are now processed meats that are labeled "without nitrites"; nitrites are a potential cause of cancer in humans. But if you read the ingredients, nitrites have been replaced by a celery culture, which is a nitrite that occurs naturally. Since it's still a nitrite, don't be fooled and avoid these processed meats.

Chapter 5: Your Intestinal Tract and Multiple sclerosis

Intestinal flora is composed of an astounding number of bacteria; 500 to 1,000 species live in the body of an individual. There are around 100 trillion bacteria in the gut, 10 times more than the number of cells in the entire body (Hyman, 2013). On average, these bacteria weigh three pounds and they are essential in balancing the immune system.

How friendly bacteria protect us

This complex, friendly bacterial flora helps in food digestion and protects us against harmful parasites, viruses, yeasts and bacteria—like the potentially deadly C difficile. Growth of these harmful microorganisms is usually limited when beneficial bacterial families are already present. C difficile can cause major health problems, like diarrhea or demineralization, when intestinal flora is decimated by antibiotics, which destroy friendly bacterial flora. Yeast can also grow exponentially when intestinal flora is decimated, resulting in *Candida albicans*, a yeast overgrowth condition that damages the intestinal lining and makes the patient very sensitive to sugars, alcohol, vinegar and fermented foods

(Martin, 2000). For these reasons, it's important to maintain good bacterial flora, or to take steps to rebuild it if it's damaged. When friendly bacteria are healthy, they can produce by-products like short-chain fatty acids that effectively reduce inflammation in the body (Hyman, 2013).

Missing Bacteria

Researchers have found that depression sufferers are missing certain types of friendly bacteria in their gut, among them Coprococcus and Dialister. These friendly bacteria produce butyrate molecules in the gut, which is a powerful anti-inflammatory agent (Guillemette, 2019). So, if you are missing these bacteria, your gut is producing inflammatory molecules that will enter your blood stream and reach different part of your body, possibly triggering multiple sclerosis.

How bad bacteria create disease

An unbalanced, low-fiber diet can cause bad bacteria to multiply and produce by-products that create inflammation and trigger asthma, eczema and allergies. Diseases that seem unrelated to the gut are, in fact, directly related to gut health. Therefore, patients with colitis can also have inflamed joints because all inflammation takes root in the gut and then spreads.

Our gut and mental health

Even patients without problematic gut symptoms who are treated for gut issues get relief from their asthma, headaches, acne, attention deficit, depression—and yes, multiple sclerosis. Some patients with delirium can be cured by taking antibiotics that kill toxic bacteria in the gut (Hyman, 2013); bacteria can affect mental health because of the toxins they produce. Children with autism can also have their condition improved significantly when given probiotics (Permutter, 2015), which are good bacteria that protect our intestinal lining.

The proverb, "you are what you eat," dating from the ancient Greeks, is so true when it comes to bacteria in the gut. Eating wholesome and healthy fresh foods helps good bacteria multiply. In contrast, eating processed, low-fiber foods allows bad bacteria to take over, producing toxins that create inflammation in the entire body which can result in many forms of disease and mental illness.

The intestinal lining

The lining of the intestine is a barrier between the outside world and your inner body. It's the last line of defense against potentially harmful bacteria, the most important filter the body has. This barrier should only allow through the basic molecules we need to maintain energy, and vitamin and mineral levels. Carbohydrates and complex sugars are broken down into simple sugars, and proteins into amino acids. When the body must deal with larger molecules that have not been broken down properly by enzymes, the intestinal lining can become clogged so that the larger molecules accumulate and can't be absorbed or eliminated sufficiently to maintain healthy gut function.

When the gut barrier fails

The intestinal lining is thin; it consists of one layer of enterocyte cells. This is all there is that protects us from the outside world. Normally, this lining protects us from foods that are not sufficiently broken down; but when these bigger food molecules occur in ever-increasing numbers, the barrier function fails. The accumulation of large molecules in the intestinal tract favors putrefaction and the growth of harmful bacteria that, over time, will attack the intestinal lining and make small perforations. These large molecules then leak into the blood stream. This condition is referred to as a "permeable lining" or "leaky gut." (TROTTER, 2015)

The inflammation reaction to food

These large, alien food molecules are then attacked by the immune system, sending cytokines in our blood to try to kill the invaders, creating inflammation, allergies, multiple sclerosis and a variety of other diseases. The immune system has can tolerate certain larger food molecules if their numbers are limited, but it reacts strongly causing allergies and inflammation when the number of invading molecules is excessive. You can also develop milk, eggs or gluten intolerances, for example, or intolerance to any food that the body reacts to as an invader. Medications like aspirin, ibuprofen (Advil) and antibiotics can also have a damaging effect on the gut lining.

Multiple sclerosis sufferers have leaky guts

Most inflammatory disease sufferers have a permeable bowel or leaky gut that lets undigested food molecules into the blood stream. The immune system then attacks the body—instead of protecting it—while trying to kill the undigested and foreign invaders. This is an autoimmune disorder that affects millions.

The direct link between food and inflammation

The Japanese people exemplify how the food we eat affects inflammatory diseases through the process described above. Before 1970, when they ate a traditional Japanese diet of primarily rice and vegetables, Japanese people had virtually no inflammatory diseases. Since they have adopted a westernized diet that includes grains and milk products, they have experienced the rapid growth of inflammatory diseases. The same can be said about other societies around the world that have recently adopted similar westernized dietary changes; the Innus have also experienced a rapid increase in autoimmune disorders.

The damage can be reversed

Fortunately, the damage inflicted by these foods can be reversed if they are withdrawn from your diet. Gluten intolerance is the best example. When gluten is completely withdrawn, the damaged intestinal tract heals and regains its normal state after four to six months, and it stays healthy if gluten is not reintroduced into the diet. The same can be said about other inflammatory diseases like multiple sclerosis; if the food that causes inflammation is withdrawn, the inflammation will permanently disappear. But even a small amount of that food can trigger inflammation, causing symptoms to return. The immune system remembers these food invaders and is ready to attack them when they are reintroduced. Staying inflammation-free is a lifelong commitment.

Antibiotics

There is evidence that some antibiotics can relieve depression symptoms, but not as a long-term solution. If an antibiotic helps in the short term, it's because it has killed certain bad bacteria which produce toxins that create inflammation. But these toxins and bad bacteria exist in the first place as the result of the unbalanced gut flora where bad bacteria have taken over. They have done so due to an insufficient amount of fiber in the diet as well as all the refined foods consumed every day. An antibiotic will aggravate the problem over a longer period because it will kill *all* bacteria—the bad and the good—leaving the gut without protection against destructive bacteria like C difficile, which kills thousands of patients every year.

When antibiotics are taken over an extended period, irritable bowel syndrome and food allergies can develop because the antibiotic damages the thin gut lining allowing big food molecules to enter the blood stream, which the immune system will attack, causing inflammation to resurface. Therefore, the real solution is to stay away from antibiotics and eat whole foods and plenty of fiber. Prebiotic and probiotic supplements can also help rebalance the gut.

Probiotics

Probiotics are the good bacteria the gut needs for maintaining health. There are many brands on the market but it's best to buy those that are refrigerated and that are linked to studies proving their effectiveness, such as Bio-K or Visbiome, a powerful probiotic you can ordered online. Look for the strains Lactobacillus acidophilus and Bifidobacterium bifidum—and the more strains the better. Start with a dose of 12 billion per day then move up to 25 billion per day the following week, and possibly 50 billion per day the week after if you have good results and want to see whether you can achieve even more improvement. After taking antibiotics you can even go to 100 billion per day or more to rebuild your gut flora, but make sure to increase the dose slowly. You might feel some discomfort at first as bad bacteria are killed, but this will pass. Visbiome has 450 billion probiotics per dose, a high dose capable of healing your gut.

Flora diversity is the key to health since the immune system is mainly based in the gut—to function well, it needs all those good bacteria to fight the bad bacteria. It has been proven in a study that probiotics, our friendly bacteria, can influence our brain and prevent or cure depression (Gruhier, 2015). Probiotics can do it by preventing cytokine inflammatory toxins in the gut to reach our blood and brain.

Chapter 6: Fiber

For optimal health, men should eat 38 grams of fiber and women 25 grams, but the average is around 15 grams currently (Zelman, 2020), less than half the amount needed for men. This is one of the reasons that modern humans are not absorbing or digesting food properly.

Soluble fiber is important. It can be found in the foods we eat like fruits, but we can add a diet supplement of flaxseed or psyllium powder, which are very high in soluble fiber. Psyllium powder dissolved in water becomes a gel that will aide bowel movement, ease constipation or diarrhea symptoms, control sugar levels, and act as a prebiotic that will help good bacteria flourish in the gut. Insoluble fiber from bran, whole fruits and vegetables will help produce short-chain fatty acids that the gut needs to function and repair itself. Eating more fiber, especially soluble fiber, will help eliminate toxins in the gut which, in turn, will lower inflammation in the entire body.

Fiber and the immune system

Fiber is essential for maintaining diverse intestinal flora; friendly bacteria will make the immune system much stronger and more resistant to outside invaders like harmful bacteria, yeast or fungi. Therefore, people with more diverse gut flora are better able to resist the C difficile bacteria, while hospital patients on antibiotics whose gut flora is weaker can more easily contract C difficile and can become very sick with diarrhea that can threaten their lives—all because of the lack of flora in the gut. Fiber prevents putrefaction and the toxic overload that leads to inflammation and multiple sclerosis. Eating more fiber will help eliminate inflammation.

The effects of lack of fiber

Fiber is crucial in ways we are just beginning to understand. Identical twins can be very different weights, even though they are genetically similar. One twin can be slim and the other can be overweight. The difference is the result of their intestinal flora. The twin who eats a lot of fiber will have a more diverse intestinal flora and be thin because its flora will help control weight by limiting the calories absorbed. The overweight twin who eats less fiber has a less diverse flora; the strains of the remaining flora increase the calorie intake from foods, making this twin fatter despite the same amount of food intake. Therefore, the cause is not genetic, or the amount of food eaten—how gut flora diversity reacts to foods is what can cause us to be fat or thin.

Make sure you eat enough fiber to produce a fast bowel-transit time, which prevents food putrefaction and toxins in your gut. But it must be the right kind of fiber—not fiber from wheat with its gut-irritating gluten.

How to add more fiber

When starting to eat more fiber, do it gradually to allow your gut to become used to this change of diet. If you transition too quickly you could experience cramps, which could discourage an increase in fiber intake. Add an increased amount each week over a few weeks because your gut needs weeks to adapt to a significant increase in fiber. The best natural fiber is obtained by eating more fruits and vegetables, but using a supplement can also be considered if it's difficult for you to add enough fiber.

If you start by using a flaxseed or psyllium supplement, begin slowly so your gut can get used to the change. For example, you can take a half teaspoon once each day the first week; then take a full teaspoon each day the second week. Take the supplement with juice if you don't like its taste or use half water and half juice to lower your sugar intake. It's essential to drink a full glass of water with the full teaspoon of psyllium or flaxseed supplement because both absorb lots of water. Liquid is needed to move the gel mixture through the bowel—not enough liquid will result in constipation. Drinking more water throughout the day will also help your bowel movement if you use psyllium supplements.

Prebiotic fiber

Prebiotic fiber feeds the good bacteria in the gut and allows them to multiply and overtake the bad bacteria. Fructo-oligosaccharide (FOS), a sugar, and inulin are the most commonly available prebiotics. If prebiotics are combined with probiotics—the good bacteria—there will be a synergistic effect that multiplies the good bacteria. Many foods also contain prebiotic fiber including asparagus, bananas, eggplant, garlic, legumes, onions, peas, etc.

Chapter 7: It's Not Just What You Eat—
It's How You Cook It

The Maillard reactions: How grilling food increases symptoms

Toxins can be the product of the food we eat, but they also result from the way we cook our food. Everyone likes a steak cooked on the grill. Grilled and roasted meat get their taste from the Maillard reaction, when sugar and proteins fuse from the heat of the flame. This complex reaction turns the color of meat yellow-brown and results in unique aromatic flavors from the new molecules created during cooking.

At a high temperature, the reaction between amino acids (proteins) and sugars produces advanced glycation end products (AGEs), or glycotoxins, which are known to increase oxidative stress and inflammation. Grilling meat increases glycotoxins 10 to 100 times compared to uncooked or boiled meat (Uribarri, 2010). Think about it—100 times more toxins that will increase your inflammation. Carbohydrate-rich foods like vegetables and grains will create relatively few toxins even after being cooked; the major problem lies with grilled, roasted or fried meat and fatty food.

Meat must be dehydrated on the grill or in a pan for this savory reaction to occur. That is why steamed, or boiled meat has far less taste: the Maillard reaction did not occur and the savory but toxic new molecules were not created. Any dry heat applied to meat and other food will create toxins, up to 100 times more than those contained in raw or boiled foods. These elevated toxins become highly oxidative, inflammatory and pathogenic.

The following is a table showing the advanced glycation end product (AGE) content of certain foods, based on their carboxymethyl-lysine (CML) content (in kU/100 g) (Uribarri, 2010):

Fats
Butter 23,000
Margarine 17,000
Mayonnaise 9,000

Mayonnaise (low-fat) 2,000

It is clear that animal products like butter contain more glycotoxins than vegetable products such as margarine, but they are both very high in glycotoxins and should be avoided. Fat content makes a big difference in the level of glycotoxins; consider low-fat instead of regular mayonnaise to dramatically reduce the glycotoxin level contained in your food.

Liquid fats

Sesame oil 22,000

Peanut oil 11,400

Olive oil (extra virgin, first cold press) 10,000

Canola oil 9,000

Sunflower oil 3,900

Corn oil 2,500

Salad dressing (Caesar) 700

Salad Dressing (Italian) 300

Salad dressing (French) 100

Salad dressing (French lite) 0

Salad dressing (Italian lite) 0

The right choice of oil is crucial for lowering your glycotoxin level since there is up to 10 times more glycotoxin in some oils—sunflower oil is better than sesame oil. Lower-quality oils that are less expensive are usually heated more to produce higher oil output, which also raises the level of toxins in the oil. It's always better to choose extra virgin and first cold-pressed oil because it contains many fewer glycotoxins. Olive oil, a good choice for lowering cholesterol, is only average concerning glycotoxins. Sunflower oil should be the preferred choice, but make sure it's cold-pressed because heat-pressed commercial brands cause the glycotoxin level to explode.

Salad dressings are lower in glycotoxins if they contain water and vinegar with the oil; lite versions without any fat contain low glycotoxins.

Nuts

Peanut butter 7,500

Peanuts (dry roasted) 6,400

Almonds (roasted) 6,600

Sunflower seeds (roasted) 4,700

Sunflower seeds (raw) 2,500

Any high-fat roasted products, even nuts, contain a high glycotoxin level. The raw version is much better because it has half the toxins.

Meat

Beef (burger) 5,500

Beef (roast) 6,000

Grilled beef (steak) 7500

Big Mac 8,000

Beef (raw) 700

Beef (stewed) 2,000

Veggie burger (microwaved) 70

Veggie burger (cooked with spray) 149

There is a steep rise in the level of glycotoxin from raw to roasted or grilled beef. But since raw meat can carry parasites that can colonize your gut and make you sick, beef stew is the wisest option. The burgers we love so much carry a high load of glycotoxins—their good taste can translate into inflammation and distress for multiple sclerosis sufferers who indulge. Veggie versions, even cooked, are a much better choice for multiple sclerosis sufferers because they won't create inflammation.

Chicken

Chicken (roasted) 9,000

Chicken McGrill 5,000

Chicken (boiled in water) 1,000

All meat (whether beef or something else) reacts the same to dry heat, as can be seen for chicken, and there is a dramatic increase in glycotoxins compared to boiled versions.

Bacon (pan fried) 92,000

Bacon (microwaved) 9,000

Processed meats like bacon or ham carry a very high load of dangerous glycotoxins. But if you can't live without bacon, it is definitely much lower in glycotoxins heated in the microwave than when fried—fried bacon has 10 times more glycotoxins.

Fish

Salmon (raw) 500

Tuna (canned, in water) 500

Salmon (broiled) 4,500

Fish also reacts to heat; it's preferable to cook fish in a broth or sauce because the glycotoxin level will be much lower.

Dairy products

Milk (whole) 5

Yogurt (vanilla) 10

Cheese (cheddar) 5,000

Cheese (mozzarella, reduced fat) 1,500

Pizza (thin crust) 7,000

Cream cheese (Philadelphia) 8,700

Unprocessed or lightly processed milk products are low in glycotoxins, but they are suitable adult human consumption, as we have seen. As with meat, the fat content in cheese plays a large roll in how much glycotoxin it contains, and fatty cheese is the worst choice.

Tofu (sautéed) 6,000

Tofu (raw) 1,000

Tofu would seem like a safe choice because it is vegetable-based, but once it's sautéed it contains a high level of glycotoxins and is as bad as meat.

Sandwich (cheese, toasted) 4,500

Bread (100% whole wheat, toasted) 120

Bread (100% whole wheat) 75

Glycotoxins in bread double when it's toasted, but these levels are low compared to the amount contained in meat or cheese. All considered, it's much better to keep eating toasted bread than grilled meat or cheese if you want to significantly reduce your inflammation, but without sacrificing too much at once.

Wheat (puffed) 20

Corn (flakes) 250

In general, cereals have a low glycotoxin level compared to meat and cheese, even when it's toasted like corn flakes. By choosing a puffed variety, you can cut 90% more glycotoxins.

Pasta (cooked 12 minutes) 240

Pasta (cooked 8 minutes) 110

Rice (cooked 30 minutes) 10

Rice (cooked 30 minutes or pan fried 10 minutes) 30

The length of time food is cooked influences it's glycotoxin level—the glycotoxin in pasta doubles when cooked 12 minutes instead of 8 minutes. Rice is the best choice among all cereals because it maintains a low glycotoxin level no matter how it's prepared.

Potato (white, boiled 25 minutes) 20

Potato (white, roasted 45 minutes) 220

Potato (white, French fries) 1,500

Boiled potatoes are always best, roasted is still not bad, but fried potatoes are much worse because the glycotoxin explodes. French fries and potato chips are especially problematic since high levels of acrylamide, a compound that can cause cancer, form during the frying process.

Chips (corn) 500

Chips (potato) 3,000

Making the right choice in chips can make a big difference—corn chips have a much lower glycotoxin level and no acrylamide.

Cracker (rice or corn) 130

Cracker (wheat, toasted) 900

It's amazing how just the toasting operation can dramatically increase glycotoxins!

Granola bar (soft) 500

Granola bar (hard) 3,000

Cookie (chocolate chip) 1,700

Again, the hard granola bar is toasted and the soft one is made with puffed rice, which makes a world of difference in their glycotoxin levels. A chocolate chip cookie is baked but also has a lot of fat, making it a good candidate for a high level of glycotoxins—1,700 for the cookie may seem reasonable, but who can stop at *one*?

Apple 10

Apple (baked) 50

Candy (dark chocolate) 1,700

The right choice of snacks and sweets is crucial to feeling well again, and not just because of the vitamins and minerals in fruit, like a tasty apple, versus those in candy. Natural, whole food is the right choice.

Vegetables (raw carrots, celery, tomato, etc.) 10 to 40

Salad (lentil and potato) 120

Vegetables (grilled) 250

The difference between raw and grilled vegetables is the added fat that increases glycotoxins. But even grilled vegetables, with 250 glycotoxins, are far less damaging than a grilled steak, with a glycotoxin level of 7,500. If you don't want to cut out that grilled taste when you want a treat, cut out grilled meat and keep eating grilled vegetables.

Toxic molecules

The more flavor you create by grilling, roasting or toasting, the more toxic your meat and other food become. Heated animal products that are high in fat and proteins—like meat—are the worst. The longer meat is cooked and the higher the cooking temperature, the more toxins are created. Cancer molecules such as heterocyclic amines and polycyclic aromatic hydrocarbons increase when fat falls on the flame. These molecules can create cancerous mutations in DNA. Studies have shown that, in the past 15 years, consumption of polycyclic aromatic hydrocarbons affects the development of cancers in rats, including colon, prostate and breast cancer (Casgrain, 2013).

The right way to cook meat

It's preferable to cook food the least amount of time possible and at the lowest possible temperature to lower the intake of toxins and the general risk of cancer. Those who consume meat that's cooked rare (bloody in the middle) have three times fewer chances of developing stomach cancer than those who eat it well done. On the other hand, you must be careful when eating bloody meat because it can transmit intestinal parasites, especially underdone pork and chicken. It's also good to reduce your total consumption of red meat because it has been associated with colorectal cancer.

The toxic molecules that form when grilling meat at a high temperature can't be broken down by digestive enzymes and will trigger inflammatory reactions in a certain percentage of the population. It is vitally important that you stop eating grilled meat to eliminate an inflammatory disease like multiple sclerosis.

Meat that doesn't cause inflammation

The good news is that there are other ways to consume meat that is full of flavor. Meat that is boiled with spices, herbs and vegetables like carrots, celery or onion can make a delicious broth, which can then be turned into a sauce by adding rice flour blended with a whip (not wheat flour, which causes inflammation). The new flavors that are created by mixing different combinations of herbs, spices and vegetables will make the transition to boiled meat easy. If meat is boiled there is no evaporation from the surface of the food, so there is no Maillard reaction and inflammatory toxins won't be created.

Vegetables that don't cause inflammation

Steaming vegetables will not result in glycation and conserves all nutrients, vitamins and minerals. Even when cooked, all carbohydrate-rich foods like whole grains, vegetables and fruits have low levels of glycotoxins; it's best to emphasis them in your diet to keep flavor on your plate. But be sure to use the least amount of fat possible when cooking vegetables because fat has high levels of glycotoxins.

Choosing meat

At the supermarket, look for meat without antibiotics and hormones. These are now more commonly available, and usually at an affordable price. Even better is organically raised meat, which means that animals were fed pesticide-free grains—unfortunately, these can be more expensive.

Raw food

It's preferable to eat raw food because cooked food and its transformed molecules tend to trigger more reactions in the body. A research showed that animals eating raw food had much less inflammation than animals eating cooked food (Seignalet, 2012).

Preference should be given to raw fruits and vegetables, as long as they're well washed—a task for which water and brushing are not even enough because harmful bacteria, yeast and parasites can remain on surfaces, especially on vegetables that can't be brushed properly. The only way to make sure surface bacteria have been removed is to submerge fruits and vegetables in water that's mixed with a teaspoon of hydrogen peroxide for 10 minutes. Then, rinse the vegetables or fruits with fresh water.

Eating raw meat is more dangerous because bacteria and parasites can proliferate on surfaces. A piece of meat can go through many hands and the tools used for cutting are not necessarily as clean as they should be. It's preferable to cook meat minimally on the surface, either boiled or stewed, but not grilled or roasted because of the glycotoxins produced.

What about the microwave?

Cooking time in a microwave is usually short and no higher than 75 degrees Celsius, which seems better than grilling or roasting. But a microwave emits waves that change the structure of food molecules and therefore its use should be limited or avoided.

Oil

The production of oil has changed considerably since industrialization. Prior to that, oil was pressed mechanically and at a low temperature, which conserved all the essential fats—but only 30% of the oil could be recovered from this simple process. By heating oil to 200 degrees Celsius, manufacturers could recover 70% of the oil but, of course, this came at a price. Dangerous trans fat was created with this process. For heated oil to be edible, it must go through many manipulations: refining, hydrogenation and other chemical processes, all of which change the nature of the oil and raise the glycotoxin level (Teicholz, 2014). This is how oil that triggers inflammation is produced.

Only buy oil that has been mechanically separated at low temperature, and only first-pressed oil that does not undergo any chemical processes. Only organic oil provides this level of quality.

Margarine is also heated at high temperatures and goes through different chemical processes. It should be avoided because it will trigger inflammation.

Finally, butter is made from milk products and, as such, should be avoided since the body's enzymes can't break it down properly and it also has high levels of glycotoxins.

Cholesterol

Bad cholesterol, or low-density lipoprotein (LDL), can accumulate in arteries and begin the inflammation process because it's another irritant to your system. Lowering your LDL and increasing your good cholesterol or high-density lipoprotein (HDL) will help lower inflammation.

Diet is the way to support good cholesterol; eat less saturated fat from meat and more fruits and vegetables. There are also drugs (Lipitor, etc.) that can lower the LDL level in your blood, but they must be accompanied by a healthy diet to have the desired effect.

A good way to reduce LDL is to have 1.5 tablespoons per day of olive oil with a salad or add it to any meal; this has been shown to reduce cholesterol in the arteries in one week.[12]

Sunflower or olive oil should replace butter (high in saturated fats) and margarine (processed using heat). Cold-pressed, extra virgin oil that is not heated at a high temperature—like commercially processed oil—is essential for receiving the benefits of many powerful antioxidants.

Chapter 8: Should You Switch to Organic Foods?

Organic food is increasingly popular because it does not contain pesticides, as do foods produced using conventional agricultural methods. There are more than 100 different types of agricultural pesticides in use today, and all these chemicals are harmful to our health. Most people think that washing vegetables thoroughly will remove pesticides, but that's not the case. Industrial pesticides enter the vegetables to some degree, so even well-washed or peeled, you can still be exposed to these detrimental chemicals. In addition, many vegetables like broccoli or grapes are hard to brush. Rinsing is not enough to avoid eating residual pesticides.

Vegetarians

A vegetarian diet is meatless but can still include animal milk or milk products, which our enzymes have a hard time breaking down, so vegetarian is not the way to go. Without a source of complete proteins, the body can weaken, making it more susceptible to disease. Vegetables supply incomplete proteins; even if a variety of vegetables is used to balance proteins, the amount of plant-based protein one can eat is insufficient for the body's needs. Also, I have seen vegetarians develop colon cancer, which makes no sense because it's supposed to be a healthier way of eating. However, if you don't eat organic foods you are consuming a lot more fruits and vegetables that have been spayed repeatedly with pesticides that can cause this type of cancer.

Vegans

A vegan diet is even riskier because it includes no animal proteins at all, not even milk or eggs, so the risk of a protein deficiency is high. The body needs protein for almost every one of its tasks, like constructing muscle tissue or making antibodies for the immune system. Bodies require a steady intake of protein each day because they can't store proteins. And, if a vegan diet is not organic, pesticide intake will be dangerously high.

Some multiple sclerosis sufferers find that certain proteins can trigger inflammation, and a diet without milk, eggs, meat or animal products can significantly reduce their level of inflammation. If you try everything suggested in this book and still have symptoms, an animal product-free diet can be worth trying out for one month to see if there is improvement.

The problem with vegetable proteins

Vegetable proteins are incomplete because they are missing an essential amino acid. For example, the lysine or leucine in grains is insufficient; to be complete, these must be complemented with soy or lentils in high amounts. But many people cannot tolerate soy, or will develop an intolerance over time, so it's not a good long-term solution for soy to be the source of your complete proteins if your body reacts to it. And it's hard to eat enough vegetable proteins to supply the body's needs—it's a risky regime that can do more harm than good.

Pesticide use

Another problem with industrial agriculture is the amount of pesticide it applies to our food. An apple can be sprayed 10 to 15 times throughout a season—that's 10 to 15 layers of pesticide added to the apple you eat. If the general public was aware of this, many would reject conventional agriculture. Because we don't *see* it and are told by the industry that the amount of pesticide use is within acceptable limits, most accept that message on faith, which they should not do. You would never spray the vegetables in your garden once or twice a week to maturity—you would be afraid to eat them.

And yet we accept this from the agricultural industry because we don't actually see it. Eating organic produce allows you to avoid a multitude of pesticide showers on your vegetables.

In many countries, the country of origin of ingredients is not disclosed, adding to the problem. For example, apple juice can be packaged in your own country, but the apple concentrate originated in China where they use toxic pesticides that are banned in Western countries, and we end up eating or drinking these products because the origin of the ingredient is hidden. When you buy organic products, certification of the food you buy eliminates the problem because all ingredients are verified as organic in their country of origin, making sure organic practices are applied.

Oversight of pesticide use

It might surprise you how little oversight there is to control the amount of pesticides the agricultural industry actually uses. Only a fraction of products get tested—and they're only tested for certain pesticides, but not for the many others available for use. Western countries have regulations, but they are often not followed because of the lack of oversight.

Now imagine the situation in Third World countries where there is little or no regulation. Those countries use pesticides that are extremely toxic, which end up in the food on our plates after traveling halfway around the world. They even use larger amounts of pesticides—pesticides that have been proven to cause cancer. Western countries ban those from their soil, but we still are exposed to them in our food when it is imported from Third World countries. Big corporations only care about profits, not your health.

There are countless cases of agricultural workers developing different types of cancer after spraying pesticides on crops. The cancer rate of these workers is much higher than among the general population, alarming us to the fact that these pesticides are toxic to one's health.

Look in your supermarket cart next time you're shopping. The percentage of fruits and vegetables coming from Third World countries is high—you will be shocked by how much we depend on them for our food supply. All these non-organically grown fruits and vegetables are contaminated by toxic pesticides, some of which are banned in Western countries.

Safety of pesticides

The most-used herbicide in the world, glyphosate (commercially known as Round Up), can kill the weeds in your yard and is used on more than 50% of all crops in the world such as corn, soy, wheat or canola. It has been deemed safe to use, mostly by the manufacturer's studies that are biased in the interest of declaring it safe so they can sell it. Often these studies are not made public, so they cannot be scrutinized by the scientific community. Even more troubling, when glyphosate is blended with other chemicals, as it is in eight of the nine most-used brands on the market, the result can be up to 1,000 times more toxic that glyphosate alone (Mesly, 2017).

All existing studies have been done on glyphosate alone—but we eat food treated with blended chemicals that are up to 1,000 times more toxic than glyphosate alone, which makes that food a high cancer risk to humans. There is no safe amount of exposure when a chemical is so toxic. The International Cancer Research Center, linked to the World Health Organization, declared in 2015 that glyphosate is a probable cause of cancer in humans.

Glyphosate has been proven to be toxic in high concentrations; the question remains, how toxic is it if taken in small amounts over an extended period? In 2017, California added glyphosate to its list of potentially carcinogenic products. Other states are still deliberating the issue. The safest approach is to buy organic products to avoid the problem.

Glyphosate is even used to kill off the plants when harvesting, which dries cereals more quickly—that is how abusive the use of these pesticides has become. According to endocrinologist Zach Bush, in *GMO Revealed*, the abuse is responsible for the epidemic of celiac disease, a severe intolerance to gluten. Many of his patients experience improved health when they start eating organic products.

A *green* food label is not enough—the agricultural industry uses green-label marketing to fool customers into believing they are buying organic when they are not. Buy only products that are labeled *organic* by a third-party certification organization that is recognized internationally.

Vegetarians and pesticides

There is a growing number of vegetarians who develop colorectal cancer. This often comes as a shock to vegetarians who thought their diets would protect them from this type of cancer—they avoided meat, which they thought was its source. But the answer lies elsewhere. Vegetarians' colorectal cancer is caused by eating more vegetables—supposedly good for one's health—but actually exposes them to higher levels of pesticide intake. The pesticide-ladened vegetables they eat are making them sick.

The cost of organic food

There is a higher cost to eating organic food since a bigger part of the crop is lost to insects as well as fungi or bacterial plant diseases. But as organic agriculture becomes more mainstream and organic products are now available in conventional supermarkets, the cost is coming down as the sales volume goes up. Ultimately, the higher cost of eating organic food can save or extend your life because you won't develop cancer. Eating food contaminated by harmful pesticides is not even an option for me, so think of it as the price you pay to eat healthy food, and never again worry about pesticides.

Other advantages to organic food

Organic products contain fewer additives when they are processed; their ingredients list is much shorter, simpler and usually contains natural and real products, not industrially created chemicals. By eating processed organic products, you will avoid additives that can trigger an arthritic inflammatory reaction. Never eat a processed product that has ingredients you don't understand—when you eat it your body won't be able to recognize them either. When an ingredient is identified as foreign, your immune system will try to attack it, causing inflammation. For example, I like to eat apple jelly on toast for breakfast. The brand I buy only has apples and sugar listed as ingredients—that's it! Other brands have a long list of ingredients and some of them are chemicals that I don't want in my body.

Pesticides are recognized as being a source of cancer in humans but also are responsible for other diseases. They can trigger inflammatory reactions in the body that can result in multiple sclerosis, even when present at only trace levels. All non-organic vegetables, especially those that are difficult to brush, should be avoided completely by multiple sclerosis sufferers.

Organic meat

If you want to go commit completely, you can expand your organic intake to other products including meat, which is more expensive since the animals are fed organic grains. Non-organic meat is raised using industrial farming methods—animals can be fed with reprocessed animal carcasses and chemical additives. Antibiotics are also used to make these animals grow faster, which is unnatural and harmful. This practice has caused the build-up of antibiotic resistance around the world, and the result is that thousands of people die every year. We are losing the battle against bacteria, which have learned to adapt to antibiotics used to kill them.

Our hospitals are now struggling with these super bacteria that can resist the most powerful antibiotics. The irresponsible practices of the meat industry are largely responsible for this crisis that will affect us all.

How organic can be affordable

If eating organic meat is too expensive for your budget, at least start eating organic vegetables and fruits—that change will result in a huge health gain. You can also buy meat that's from animals raised without antibiotics or hormones. These are less expensive than organic products and better than standard meat. An even better approach would be to eat less meat; then the money saved can be spent on organic meat.

GMO

Genetically modified organisms (GMOs) are another problem because many countries don't require manufacturers to inform consumers that a product has been genetically modified. There are now varieties of corn, wheat and soy, to name only a few, that are genetically modified to resist glyphosate. These crops can be sprayed repeatedly—every week—with glyphosate so that they contain a high level of this herbicide, yet they can be sold without informing consumers on product packaging. They can even be labeled *healthy* and *natural* products at the supermarket even though they are sprayed continuously with pesticides or herbicides, which are not natural at all.

The gene modifications created artificially in a lab result in new molecules that, again, the body lacks the enzymes to digest properly. The best way to avoid genetically modified products is to eat those that are organic because, for organic agricultural products, it is forbidden to use GMOs.

A two-year study (the usual study length is 3 months), from 2012, by researcher Gilles-Eric Seralini, found tumors on mice that ate GMO corn, as well as liver and renal problems. These mice died prematurely. GMO manufacturers have tried in multiple ways to discredit this study but have failed so far— another reason to switch to organic products since they must not contain any GMOs.

Plants are now genetically modified to be glyphosate resistant or "ready" so that they can be treated over and over again with chemicals that KILL every other living plant around it. If glyphosate can kill all plant life, how can it not be harmful to humans? The manufacturers of glyphosate and some governments say it's a question of dosage. If your vegetables are sprayed every week with herbicides all summer long, do you still feel safe eating them? GMO plants repeatedly sprayed with glyphosate strongly correlate with the increase in diabetes, Alzheimer's disease, autism and thyroid problems (Seneff, 2019).

Chapter 9: The Water You Drink

Governments tell us tap water is safe to drink, but conventional chlorine disinfection methods do not destroy everything during treatment. With today's advanced instruments, scientists are able to detect and measure the most widely-used medications—like antibiotics or antidepressants, BPA, domestic-use cleaners, microscopic plastic particles (Kinnard, 2016), and the list goes on. Residuals from women's oral contraceptives that release estrogen are creating reproductive problems for fish. This is the water our governments tell us is safe to drink.

Conventional water treatment cannot eliminate such small molecules and there are no official limits established for these water contaminants. Instead, the dilution principle is used: the residual amount should be insignificant but many of these substances—like estrogen, even in small amounts— remain active.

If you drink tap water, make sure the water treatment facility serving your area is equipped with an ozone disinfection installation. This type of treatment eliminates hormones, bacteria, viruses and most pharmacologic substances.

Ozone is a powerful disinfectant capable of eliminating molecules that resist conventional treatments. On contact with ozone, organic matter is oxidized; bacteria and viruses are killed or become inactive. Ozone also eliminates odors and bad taste.

Water treatments for safe drinking water

If ozone-treated tap water is not available in your area, and it probably isn't, I recommend adding a reverse osmosis system at home that connects to your water supply. The system must meet the NSF/ANSI 58 STANDARD for water purity. The osmosis filter has micro-pores that let water filter through, but not contaminants and bacteria. They usually use multiple stages of filtration; each stage purifies and removes larger molecules until the final elimination stage which is done by the osmosis filter.

The following are the elimination rates of a reverse osmosis system, based on the manufacturer's test results:

Bacteria and viruses, 99+%

Cryptosporidium parasites, 99%

Giardia, 99%

Protozoa parasites, 99%

Ameobic cyst parasites, 99%

Detergent, 97%

Lead, 98%

Herbicides and pesticides, 97%

Keep in mind that a reverse osmosis filter takes out all that's bad in water, but it also removes good things, including dissolved minerals such as magnesium or potassium that the body needs to function properly.

The following shows the average elimination rates of minerals using a reverse osmosis system:

Calcium, 96%

Magnesium, 96%

Potassium, 96%

Therefore, you will need an alkaline pH mineralization filter. Using mineral stone, it replaces healthy minerals that were removed during the reverse osmosis process including ionized calcium, magnesium, sodium and potassium. It also improves the pH value of water produced by the reverse osmosis process, which can be slightly acidic.

If you want an even better elimination rate, you can add a UV light filter to your reverse osmosis system. The UV light kills bacteria, viruses, and other microorganisms by interfering with their DNA. With this final step, your water will be totally safe, even if it comes from a well.

Water quality and inflammation

So why make sure the water you drink is pure? Because all the leftover molecules could potentially make your immune system react, causing inflammation. You will be healthier when you keep harmful chemicals out of your body.

Reverse osmosis systems are relatively inexpensive; they range from $200 to $500 depending on the number of stages of filtration, or if it has a pump that forces water through the reverse osmosis filter, which makes it more effective. These prices are for kits ordered on the Internet that you install yourself. Installation can take three to four hours initially, but you will save hundreds of dollars compared to having it installed by a local store. It's time well spent because you will understand how your system works. I ordered and installed an iSpring system myself, and I'm very satisfied with it. But any other NSF/ANSI-approved system will do. This system will last many years if the filters are changed every six months. That's very inexpensive for such high-quality water.

Replacement filters will cost about $50 each if you change them yourself, which takes about 30 minutes. Having them changed by a local supplier of filters is way more expensive, about $200 each. It's easy to change the filter by yourself to save money.

One thing is for sure, it's way less expensive than buying bottled water, which is not that safe anyway since limited testing is done to verify its quality. There have been recalls of bottled water because of contamination—showing that there's no purity guarantee with bottled water, regardless of what the advertisement wants us to believe. Water sources are no longer pristine; human pollution has reached every corner of the earth. But reverse osmosis will mechanically remove these contaminants for you—with bottled water there are no guaranties, the quality can be inferior to tap water...

Avoid plastic bottles

The plastic used for clear water bottles leaks microscopic plastic molecules in the water. BPA is one example, but other molecules can now be measured. If you drink water from a plastic bottle daily, the residual amount will add up over time and potentially trigger your immune system to react with inflammation. Fill-up glass bottles are now available in sports stores. Glass is much safer than plastic; it won't leak molecules into your water.

PH and multiple sclerosis

To function well, the human body needs to maintain an acid-base balance. When this is out-of-balance, diseases can occur.

Acids

We are all familiar with an acidic taste. Acids liberate corrosive hydrogen ions in water. A coin in a glass of cola will have a corroded surface within a few days; a piece of meat in cola will dissolve in a few days. Acids can burn and dissolve human tissue. Many foods don't taste acidic, but when digested are acidifying for the body because they liberate low levels of acid in the body, but on an on-going basis.

Bases

Bases liberate little or no hydrogen, which gives foods a smooth taste. All colored and green vegetables are alkaline (base) as well as potatoes, almonds, bananas, etc. Bases contain minerals like calcium or magnesium and these minerals can neutralize acids.

pH

The acidity or alkalinity of any food or chemical is measured by pH, which means the *potential* (p) to liberate *hydrogen* (H) ions. The scale measuring pH ranges from 1 to 14. A balanced or neutral pH is 7 on the pH scale. Strangely, the more acidic a substance is, the lower it scores on the scale, ranging from 6.9

to 0. Alkalinity ranges from 7 to 14. It is a logarithmic scale, so each unit is 10 times more acidic or alkaline than the previous number. Therefore, between 7 and 5 on the pH scale is 100 times more acidic.

The body's optimal pH is 7.4, or slightly alkaline (SULLIVAN, 2020).

Modern foods are too acidic

Modern processed foods are mostly acidic foods, and so is our daily food intake: meat and poultry, cereal, pasta, bread, sweets, cola, fruit juice, cheese, alcohol, coffee, etc. (Thompson, 2019). Our acidic food intake is so high that we would have to eat a colossal amount of vegetables to balance the pH, and that's impossible.

Consequences of an acid surplus

The body tries to eliminate an acid surplus through the skin (perspiration) and the kidneys (urine), but that's insufficient. Like a base that neutralizes an acid to make a neutral salt, the body uses the minerals in the system to neutralize acid, which gradually reduces the calcium, magnesium, potassium and other essential minerals in the body. This process weakens the body and opens the door to diseases.

When the body doesn't have a sufficient amount of minerals to counter acid, the acid surplus irritates tissues and creates inflammation (Vasey, 2008). The most visible signs of acid surplus are skin related: eczema, redness and itching appear. Others suffer from irritable bowels, colitis and other bowel inflammation diseases.

Anxiety is also common among those who are demineralized because magnesium and other alkaline minerals calm the nervous system.

How to eliminate acid surplus

Eating more alkaline foods like vegetables, potatoes and bananas will help maintain better pH balance. But in many cases, that will be insufficient to reverse the damage already done. To boost your alkaline intake, you can buy alkaline water at the supermarket—but it is very expensive, high in sodium and creates plastic pollution. The most efficient solution is to take a liquid alkaline mineral supplement, which has highly concentrated magnesium or potassium. Just add a few drops to a glass of water and the water will go from 7 to 8 on the pH scale; slightly alkaline water that will help reduce an acid surplus and heal inflamed membranes in the body. The goal is to reach a balance, as too much alkaline drops could create other problems like a lack a stomach acidity or kidney problems. If you buy a pH tester (about $10), you will be able to measure the change from 7 to 8 on the pH scale.

These liquid alkaline mineral supplements can be bought at any natural food store, vitamin store or through the Internet. They are called "pH drops" or "alkaline drops." After neutralizing excess acid, alkaline drops will re-mineralize your body.

These are a few commercial brands of liquid alkaline drops that can be found and ordered through the Internet or get them in a store selling natural products: Alkazone, Alkavision, Mega-Mag or Trace Minerals. Some, like Alkazone, have more potassium; others, like Mega-Mag, have more magnesium. These mineral liquids are very effective in re-mineralizing the body, much more than pills that contain bigger molecules which are harder to assimilate. If you insist on pills or caplets, use the citrate type rather than the carbonate type that is poorly absorbed by the body. But liquid minerals are best.

Positive results can be noted after a few weeks—that's the amount of time needed by the body to eliminate the acid surplus and re-mineralize itself. Once your mineral supply is back to an optimal level, the healing process can begin. When you are feeling better, you must keep using the pH drops because, if you stop, all the symptoms and the acid surplus will return.

Achieving balance in the body's pH and mineral level is the basis for starting to heal. Some experience a big improvement in the way they feel by following these simple recommendations.

Chapter 10: Other Habits to Consider

Vitamin D for multiple sclerosis

There is a link between multiple sclerosis and a low level of vitamin D. People living in northern countries where there is less daylight have a higher rate of multiple sclerosis. The body uses vitamin D to produce cathelicidins; some of which act as hormones with antibacterial and antiviral properties that sterilize toxins. Women who take a vitamin D supplements have a 40% lower risk of developing multiple sclerosis (Blum, 2013). Taking vitamin D is therefore essential for the improvement of multiple sclerosis sufferers

Chlamydia pneumoniea

When a bacteria like *C. pneumoniea* is present in the cerebrospinal fluid, as found in many multiple sclerosis patients, vitamin D will not be enough to get rid of the infection. An antibiotic such as minocycline will then be necessary (Blum, 2013) to cure the underlying infection.

Get tested for intestinal parasites

If you also suffer from digestive issues, get tested for intestinal parasites. Parasites produce toxins that can create inflammation in different parts of the body, including the brain.

You can be infected with intestinal parasites by drinking tap water. In 1993, 400,000 Milwaukee, Wisconsin, residents were infected by cryptosporidium in the city's drinking water. This is one of many cases when municipal water was not safe to drink. Approximately 28% of drinking water samples tested in the United States have been found to be contaminated with microorganisms (Lecavalier).

Water treatment plants rely on chlorine to disinfect water. This is effective in killing bacteria but not certain parasites like giardia or cryptosporidium, which can survive up to a year in water (Bueno, 1996). Bottled water is not a better choice because it is often untreated. The only way to protect oneself is to use a reverse-osmosis system at home. When away from home, choose vapor-distilled bottled water.

You can also get intestinal parasites by swimming in a lake and swallowing drops of water. Over 80% of surface water samples in the United States were found to be contaminated with microorganisms (Rose, 1990). Swimming pools, especially public ones, can have traces of feces from baby diapers that can make someone sick.

You can also be infected by parasites when eating raw fruits and vegetables that are inadequately washed and that retain parasite cysts. If you eat outdoors, be aware that flies are notorious for depositing parasite cysts when they land on food. Raw meats (steak tartare) or those that are cooked rare can put you at risk for beef and pork tapeworms. Raw or undercooked fish such as sushi or cold-smoked salmon can also carry tapeworms. Always wash your hands after handling raw meat or fish.

Pets can also transmit parasites; their fur may carry eggs or cysts picked up while rolling on the ground in backyards, sandboxes and playgrounds, or on carpets, etc. You should always wash your hands after every contact with a pet. At day care centers, diaper changing also carries the risk of parasite transmission. Any sexual practice involving anal contact puts you at risk. International travel is high-risk, too; you can be infected by a parasite from an ice cube in a drink or when you take a shower with inadequately treated water. Never drink tap water when you travel.

Parasite testing

Parasites are hard to find in stool tests. A physician will conclude you don't have a parasite after a negative stool test—but it can take 10 to 20 tests to find parasites in stool samples. Often, laboratory technicians are not trained well enough to identify parasites. Look for a lab that specializes in parasite testing and be prepared to do multiple tests before receiving a positive result. Parasites are more easily found in intestinal mucus rather than in stool; a rectal swab (a disposable anoscope is inserted into the rectum) has a much better chance of confirming the presence of a parasite.

Parasite treatment

If a parasite is identified, antibiotics will usually be prescribed by your doctor. Antibiotic treatment will make you feel better in a few days. If your stool test or tests were negative and you don't have the will or finances to pay for more tests or to travel to a center that does a rectal swab, you can try herbs that have been found to be effective and which may help in treating against parasites. Artemisia annua is the most effective herb available and can easily be found in supplement form on the internet. The Allergy Research Group, a trusted brand, offers the product Artemisinin, which is the active component of artemisia. Grapefruit seed extract is safe and can be taken over several months, the amount of time required to eliminate a parasite like giardia (Goldberg, 1998). Taking a strong and proven probiotic like Visbiome with Lactobacillus acidophilus and Bifidobacterium for at least 12 weeks can prove more effective than antibiotics for treating parasites. Using this method, Dr. Chaitow reported an 80% success rate for seriously ill people afflicted with parasites (Goldberg, 1998).

Smoking

We all know that smoking tobacco is bad; it can cause lung cancer and a variety of other diseases including heart attack. Smoke contains many irritant chemicals that can trigger inflammation. The toxic load of cigarettes is high because all these harmful chemicals, including nicotine, enter the body—not just the lungs. It is essential to stop smoking to get rid of inflammation.

Fasting

If you want proof that the food you eat is causing your multiple sclerosis, try fasting for a week and you should see remarkable effects—your inflammation will greatly diminish simply because the sources of inflammation have been removed. This is a radical measure that is hard to apply when you have a full-time job and need energy to function. But it could be considered if you take a week off work and are supervised by a health professional to get enough liquids and minerals.

Protein-free diet

A less radical way to have a fast decrease of inflammation is to follow a protein-free diet, focusing for a week on foods like rice, potatoes, fruits and vegetables. This will give you the energy needed to function, and you will be able to work, but you should still see a significant decrease in your inflammation. Why proteins? Some proteins can trigger inflammation, especially when grilled or dry roasted.

Your environment

The environment in which you work or live can also trigger inflammation. Buildings with sealed windows and central air conditioning often have poor air quality and little fresh air. The trapped air in these buildings is filled with a variety of volatile chemical contaminants that come from the carpet, paint or cleaning products. Your home can also be a problem for the same reasons.

All of these air contaminants create respiratory inflammation resulting in coughing, nasal congestion and other related problems. But they can also trigger internal inflammation when the body breathes these toxic chemicals. The glue in laminated floors or the foam in your bed can emit volatile chemicals, too. These are more expensive changes and can be considered if all else fails. If you decide to renovate, consider hard wood floors a better health choice. Choose a leather sofa instead of a fabric one--leather doesn't carry mites, dust or other allergens that can trigger inflammation and it can be easily washed, like bed linen.

Consider using a natural antiperspirant; conventional ones contain aluminum that's absorbed by your skin—yet another chemical the body can do without to prevent inflammation.

A safer environment

Use low VOC (volatile organic compounds), water-based paints and avoid carpets altogether. Gas stoves should be avoided—they release contaminants into the air. Check for mold in your home; it grows in humid, dark areas and releases spores that can cause reactions such as inflammation. Homes should not exceed 50% humidity, or a mold problem can occur. A humidity meter bought at a hardware store will help monitor the humidity level in your home; a dehumidifier can resolve a humidity problem. Remember that anything synthetic in your environment can release volatile chemicals that you can react to with inflammation, so take time to review your surroundings to identify potential problems.

Cleaning products

We like cleaning products that are smelly—we think things are cleaner when there's a strong smell. But these smells are volatile chemicals that you breathe. Any fragrance or perfume can do harm, even those in air fresheners.

Getting rid of all strong, harmful cleaning products and choosing nontoxic cleaners that contain natural essential oils are imperative. These can be found in stores selling healthier products and sometimes in mainstream supermarkets. Natural products, preferably without any perfume, can be used for kitchen surfaces, floors, washing clothes, etc.

Avoid products with bleach or ammonia. You don't need these harmful chemicals to have a clean home. Windows should be open for fresh air when using any cleaning product. And we now know that a little dirt is good for the gut microbiome. The gut needs bacteria to be healthy, so cleaning less can be a good and safe thing to do.

There has been an explosion of asthma and food allergies in kids while we have tried to keep everything bacteria-free. A lack of bacteria results in less-diverse gut flora; this weakens an immune system that treats good bacteria as an enemy because they are not recognized by the immune system. Now, some immune systems even react to safer products because of our obsession with cleanliness.

Toxin-free body products

Almost all products we buy for personal care—from toothpaste to hand cream—include chemicals that can trigger inflammatory reactions. Visit www.ewg.org to find safer choices and to see how the products you use are rated. This can make a big difference in your fight against inflammation. The strong cleaning chemicals in your toothpaste could be making you sick when you swallow some after rinsing. And imagine all the chemicals your skin absorbs while rubbing in hand cream!

Glass containers

I use glass containers to store food; avoid plastic containers— they release plastic molecules into your food. At the supermarket, choose brands using glass containers rather than plastic packaging.

Air purifiers

Using an air purifier is a good idea; it will rid all contaminants from the air. Choose a brand with a HEPA or charcoal-activated filter that can remove almost all chemicals and mold spores.

Stress

Any stress you feel inside your body should be dealt with. If your gut is tense on a regular basis, your body is in alert mode and you are not digesting your food properly. In this state, your immune system will react more intensely with inflammation.

We all spend way too much time worrying about things that may or may not happen. We just need to focus on the moment and deal with the future when it happens. If you can't do it on your own, consider the help of a psychologist or other professional. When I was younger, I had anxiety issues, but a hypnotherapist really helped me—by communicating with my *subconscious* mind, the hypnotherapist was able to reach me through messages that I was not able to access myself by talking directly to a psychologist.

I used to be really stressed at school and work, always worried about deadlines and consequences. Then, with hypnotherapy, I finally accepted different principles: "I can work calmly and finish on time," or "As long as I do my best, everything will be OK." Without hypnotherapy these mantras were ineffective, but they became a reality for me after a few sessions of deep concentration through hypnosis—then I wondered why I was so stressed before. It made all the difference in the world. Trust in your ability to adapt and let go! But use a hypnotherapist or psychologist who uses hypnosis to help you if it's not possible on your own. Taking things less seriously in general also helps.

Meditation

One of the best ways to reduce stress is to practice meditation. Simply concentrating on breathing for 10 to 15 minutes per day and feeling the air slowly flowing in and out eases tension throughout the body. Another effective technique you can try is breathing in for 5 seconds, holding your breath for another 5 seconds, and breathing out for up to 8 seconds. Doing this for 5 minutes twice a day will calm your mind. If thoughts intrude during meditation, you can repeat the mantra "I am calm."

Yoga

For some people, meditating is difficult because they fall asleep or their mind is constantly invaded by thoughts that break the calming process of meditation. Yoga is the perfect solution for resolving these issues—yoga is meditation in motion. I practice yoga and I guarantee you won't fall asleep doing these poses because they require effort. You will be focused on executing different positions and maintaining them, so it will be harder for your mind to wander off.

Yoga will strengthen and stretch your muscles, massage your internal organs and calm your nervous system. Yoga is an ancient practice but, in our modern lives, relieving tense muscles after working all day—often sitting in the same position—is extremely important; human physiology requires walking and movement.

Stand up!

A few years ago, I bought a worktable that can be raised so that I can work at my computer standing up. What a difference it made! My back stopped aching and I was less stressed when working because I don't like sitting for hours. I now usually work standing up for an hour, lower the table and work sitting down for 15 minutes to rest, then move it back up again for another hour. I have more energy at the end of my day after working in a standing position than when I'm sitting down all day.

Yes, a stand-up table has a cost, but it's an investment that will pay off in health benefits for the rest of your life. And why not ask your employer to buy you one for the office? In an age in which employers are trying to keep their employees happier and more productive, you might be surprised—they could be open to the proposition when they consider that it will keep you more alert, awake and productive at work.

I even added a treadmill that I placed under my worktable. Now I can walk slowly while working, which is both energizing and relaxing. It did wonders for my sciatic nerve pain—it went away as I walked. LifeSpan and SereneLife have different treadmill models made to fit under stand-up tables.

Powerful and proven results of meditation and yoga

Meditation and yoga have been proven effective in reducing stress by multiple studies using different measurement methods. In particular, scientific measurements using 3D scans have shown that meditation or yoga can physically reduce the size of the amygdala, the region of the brain associated with the prehistoric fight-or-flight reflex and the response to stress. As the amygdala shrinks, so does the response to stress in general (Harvey, 2014). What might have bothered you in the past will no longer do so when your amygdala is smaller.

Even more powerful, meditation can put to sleep certain genes responsible for debilitating diseases such as multiple sclerosis and can also stop the progression of the disease or altogether reverse its damage (Harvey, 2014). So, if your family has a genetic predisposition to a disease, you are no longer doomed to the same fate if you are willing to make meditation and yoga an active part of your life. In addition, you can reduce or eliminate inflammation and multiple sclerosis with meditation and yoga if they are accompanied by the nutritional advice in this book.

Heal with nature

Having regular contact with nature has been proven by multiple studies to have a soothing effect on the mind and body. Richard Louv talks about a "nature-deficit disorder"— the negative conditions created by not having access to nature to calm the brain result in being more stressed, depressed, tense, heart pounding and always being tired. Studies have shown than being in a busy urban environment with concrete and car circulation leads to rumination, being angrier and having reduced attention and concentration. Being in nature does the exact opposite, helping one's mood and ability to focus better. It's better to have a short time in nature every day than a longer period once a week because the experience resets one's thoughts each day. You could call it your *Vitamin N,* for "nature," which replenishes your energy, good mood, and ability to focus and perform better at work.

The same applies to activities in general. It's better to play and have a little fun every day than to exercise once every few days. Taking a longer break for a summer vacation is also essential for allowing your brain to log off and let go of the routine stress of daily life.

Remove breast implants

All breast implants can leak silicone, which then spreads throughout the body and triggers a variety of diseases. In a study following 25,000 women, those with breast implants were found to have a 45% higher risk of developing an autoimmune disease than women without them (ROY, 2020). The same study found that up to 80% of women who have their implants removed feel an improvement in their condition after removal. For the remaining 20%, it can take much longer if the silicone has been leaking over a long period of time. Leaked silicone can be found in women's brains, nerves, and muscles.

Remove root canals if you have them

A root canal is a procedure that tries to save and maintain a dead tooth that should be removed. Modern medicine recognizes that any dead tissue must be removed because it will cause infection, which can make patients sick or kill them. Only dentists think they can get away with this.

The problem with this procedure is that the canal is impossible to clean completely—there are always bacteria that manage to get into the peripheral micro-tubing surrounding the canal, and once the canal is sealed the bacteria can proliferate and infection will set in. The body will not be able to heal the infected area since this is a dead tooth with no blood flow to clean it. This infection and bacteria will then move to other parts of the body and trigger diseases (Kulacz, 2014).

For example, researchers have linked dental infections to several types of cancer including pancreatic, lung, gastrointestinal, throat, tongue, mouth and lip, and head and neck cancers (Kulacz, 2014).Once a tooth that has had a root canal is removed, the source of infection is gone.

For a long time, root canals were considered a safe procedure because normal X-rays did not show any infection at the root canal site, mainly because the X-ray imagery was not precise enough. Now, with new 3D scanning imagery, some holistic dentists are noticing infections where root canals are located.

When the infection disappears, the inflammation disappears as well. The removal must be done by a holistic dentist who knows how to do this procedure the right way, making sure the infection is dealt with completely with an ozone treatment. There are not too many holistic dentists around, but if you do a search using the keywords "holistic dentist," hopefully you can find one within a reasonable driving distance from your area.

Many regular dentists are still doing root canals because this is what they learned in school and they are not aware of the latest developments. However, there is now overwhelming evidence that root canals cause infections. Even if some question this new knowledge, just to be on the safe side root canals should not be performed anymore since they can potentially make people sick. There are other solutions for fixing a dead tooth that are much safer.

Removing a tooth that has had a root canal is one of the most important things you can do to get a complete remission. But since the removal of a tooth that has had a root canal involves dental surgery, you will probably want to try the other measures in this book first.

Cavitation

When a tooth is removed (especially a wisdom tooth) but the periodontal ligament under the tooth is not removed, the ligament can rot causing infection in the hole that was left. This infection can then spread throughout the body causing disease and inflammation. A holistic dentist can remove this infection, making sure the cavity is filled with solid dental bone when it heals. This is done by cleaning the tooth hole and filling it with PRF, a growth factor in the blood that converts into dental bone.

Dental titanium versus ceramic implants

Titanium implants used in dentistry are also a problem because many nerves in the entire body are connected to our teeth. A metal implant interferes with these nerves and its electrical signals. Ceramic implants do not interfere like metal implants and are tolerated much better by the body. There are a few good books on the subject: *Whole-Body Dentistry*, by Mark Breiner, will open your eyes concerning this issue.

Mercury fillings: a clear link to multiple sclerosis

The immune system reacts to mercury fillings with inflammation. Dental amalgams are 45-55% elemental mercury. Mercury is very toxic and can be lethal at high doses. It's also dangerous at lower doses, in fillings, because chewing food slowly releases mercury that then spreads into the organs and body, making you sick.

Multiple sclerosis first appeared after mercury dental fillings were introduced, around 1850 (Cambayrac, 2011). This could have been a coincidence. But multiple sclerosis is rare in Japan, where mercury fillings have been banned since 1985 (Cambayrac, 2011). Close to Japan, in Australia, where mercury fillings are still used, Australians have one of the highest levels of multiple sclerosis in the world. In 1989, it was shown that multiple sclerosis patients had five to seven times more mercury in their cerebrospinal fluid than that found in the general population (Ahlrot-Westerlund, 1989). It has also been demonstrated that mercury can damage myelin and lead to multiple sclerosis (Siblerud-Kienholz, 1997). Therefore, it is crucial to remove mercury fillings to heal from multiple sclerosis.

Choose a ceramic filling when you have a cavity. If you have mercury fillings and want to have them removed, you must choose a holistic dentist who uses the Safe Mercury Amalgam Removal Technique (SMART) of the International Academy of

Medicine and Toxicology; these are guidelines for safely removing fillings. You can see safety procedures and find a SMART-certified dentist on the SMARTchoice.com website. Don't go to a regular dentist for this procedure—removing mercury fillings can make you sick because inhaling toxic vapors caused by drilling is extremely dangerous for your health.

A study has shown that multiple sclerosis patients treated with chelating injections to reduce mercury and heavy metal deposits in their bodies felt improvement after treatment (Daunderer, 1995), so there is definitely a link between mercury and multiple sclerosis.

Teeth and overall health

Some researchers think that undiagnosed dental infections can be linked to most modern diseases and can be healed when the infection is eliminated. Therefore, if you correct the different problems mentioned in the dental section, you can improve your overall health and potentially heal your multiple sclerosis completely.

Conclusion

Autoimmune diseases like multiple sclerosis are the result of a toxic overload in your body, and your immune system tries to defend itself by responding with inflammation. Toxic overload can arise from multiple sources in a daily routine, as this book has shown. To experience a significant decrease in your symptoms, the best solution is to simultaneously remove as many sources of toxicity as possible. If you try only one solution at a time, like cutting out only gluten, the toxin reduction might not be sufficient to feel a difference because the other sources of inflammation are still active. Eating the right foods and drinking alkaline water is essential for ending the inflammation and disease cycle.

It will be hard to change old habits at first, think of it as a trial and not something definitive. Once you get used to your new routine and feel symptoms going away, you won't want to go back to your old ways.

If you reintroduce sources of inflammation into your diet, the symptoms will come back—it's a lifelong commitment to staying disease-free. You must keep your new diet for at least four months because this is the length of time the body needs to evacuate toxins and remove inflammation.

A placebo effect has a healing rate of 40%, on average. This diet has a success rate of 98% for multiple sclerosis sufferers as tested by a European study (Seignalet, 2012), well above any placebo effect, prescribed medication or medical treatment. It's an effective cure if you are willing to apply it. If you do, you will soon enjoy your new disease-free life.

Appendix A

Main Foods that Trigger Inflammation (DARLNGTON, 1991)

When these foods are removed, sensitive subjects feel an improvement in their multiple sclerosis symptoms. When these foods are reintroduced, sensitive subjects feel their multiple sclerosis symptoms worsen again. It can take up to 4 months after removal to feel an improvement, especially wheat. Notice that these products come from all food groups.

Food	% of sensitive subjects
Corn	56
Wheat	54
Bacon (pork)	39
Orange	39
Milk	37
Oat	37
Rye	34
Egg	32
Beef	32
Barley	27
Cheese	24
Grapefruit	24
Tomato	20
Nuts	20
White Sugar	20
Butter	17
Lamb	17
Soy	17

Appendix B

Permitted grains and flours:
-rice
-buckwheat
-millet
-quinoa
-amaranth
-arrowroot
-teff
-coconut flour
-potato flour
-tapioca

Grains to avoid:
-wheat
-kamut
-spelt
-rye
-oat
-barley

Gluten products to avoid:

-malt, malt vinegar
-beer (made from barley or other grains)
-couscous
-bulgur
-seitan (pure wheat gluten)
-bread
-pasta
-bagels
-crackers
-cookies
-cake
-donuts
-pastries
-bran or germs from cereals

Milk products to avoid:

-milk from cow, goat, sheep or any animal
-cheese made with milk from any animal (cow, goat, etc.)
-cream
-dairy ice cream
-dairy yogurt
-any commercial product containing milk or its components, like casein or whey (many high-protein products like energy bars or liquid meal replacements contain whey)
-butter

Permitted milk substitutes:

-rice milk and products
-millet milk
-almond or other nut milk (without sugar)
-coconut milk

Milk substitutes to avoid:

-soy milk, soy cheese and other soy products

Appendix C

The cure that has a 98% success rate with multiple sclerosis based on a European study (Seignalet, 2012)

1) No milk products (cow, goat, sheep, etc.) of any kind (yogurt, cheese, butter, cream, etc.).

   Replace with plant-based milk (from rice or nuts) and cheese, or dairy-like products.

2) No grains containing gluten (wheat, kamut, spelt, rye, oat, barley) in any product (bread, pasta, cereal, beer, bagels, crackers, cookies, cake, donuts, pastries, bran, couscous, etc.). You must search the ingredients list— many industrial products contain gluten including deli meats, ground pepper, soups, soy sauce, etc.

   Only rice is allowed in any form (bread, pasta, etc.). Buckwheat, millet, quinoa, amaranth, arrowroot, coconut flour, potato flour, and tapioca can be introduced a few months after the start of the regime; they are usually well tolerated and close to their original natural state.

3) No corn or corn products.
4) Nothing cooked over 110 degrees Celsius.

   No meat that is grilled, roasted or heat-dried in anyway, and no deli meat. Meat can only be boiled in broth to avoid toxic and inflammatory advanced glycation end products (AGEs). Broth can be thickened with rice flour for flavorful sauces or stews.

5) No refined or heated oils. Oils must be cold pressed.

6) No industrially transformed products containing additives. Use organic varieties if you still buy these products; they have many fewer harmful additives. All ingredients must be whole foods, ingredients you can understand. The ingredient list should be very short.

7) No commercial sugars (including fructose, glucose, maltose, corn syrup, cane sugar, etc.) including all the transformed foods that contain added sugars. No fruit juice—sugar absorption is too quick.

8) Eat raw food as much as possible. Cooked food should be heated to the lowest temperature and shortest time possible.

All these measures will lead to a 98% multiple sclerosis cure rate if taken seriously and done rigorously. To achieve a higher percentage of healing, add these additional measures:

9) Choose organic products that are pesticide-free.

10) Add vegetable fiber—especially prebiotic fiber—to your diet to boost intestinal flora and your immune system. Eat more fruits and vegetables and add

flaxseed or psyllium powder if necessary. No bran
from wheat or other grains that contain gluten.

11) Consider taking a probiotic supplement to heal your
gut.

12) Drink water that has been purified—eliminate
chemicals like chlorine and bacteria with a reverse
osmosis system. Bottled water can contain harmful
bacteria--nothing is pristine in nature anymore;
humans have polluted every corner of our planet.

13) Make sure the pH of your drinking water is alkaline by
adding pH drops.

14) As much as possible, try to have a chemical-free
environment. For example, the air you breath should
be free of strong cleaning products. Choose natural
alternatives.

15) Practice meditation and Yoga; both are proven to
reduce stress and help healing

16) Consider removing mercury fillings that are shown to be a trigger for multiple sclerosis.

17) Take a vitamin D supplement to help remission

References

Ahlrot-Westerlund. (1989). Mercury in Cerebrospinal Fluid in Multiple Sclerosis. *Swedish Journal of Biological Medecine*, vol.1, p. 6-7.

Appleton, N. (2009). *Suicide by Sugar.* Square One Publishers, p.7.

Blum. (2013). *The Immune System Recovery Plan.* Scribner, p. 300.

Bowers, J. (2020, 06 09). *https://www.thediabetescouncil.com/how-much-sugar-is-in-popular-drinks/.* Retrieved from https://www.thediabetescouncil.com.

Brostoff, J. G. (2000). *Food Allergies and Food Intolerances.* Rochester: Healing Arts Press, p.14.

Bueno, H. (1996). Uninvited Guests. *Keats Publishings*, 8.

CALDER, P. (2017). *https://pubmed.ncbi.nlm.nih.gov/28900017/.*

Cambayrac, F. (2011). *Vérités sur les maladies émergentes.* Mosaique-santé.

Cancer.org. (2019). *https://www.cancer.org/cancer/cancer-causes/acrylamide.html.*

Casgrain. (2013, June-July). Barbecue pour le meilleur et sans le pire. *Quebec Science*, pp. 17-20.

CORDAIN, L. (2002). *The Paleo Diet.* New Jersey: John Wiley and Sons.

Darlington. (1986). *Placebo controlled, blind study of dietary manipulation therapy in rheumatoid arthritis.* Lancet, pp. 236-238.

DARLINGTON. (1991). *Diets for rheumatoid arthritis.* Lancet, pp.308, 1209.

DARLNGTON. (1991). *Diets for rheumatoid arthritis .* Lancet, 338, 1209. .

Daunderer. (1995). Les effets néfastes des amalgames, leur détection, leur thérapie. *Ecomed.*

D'souza, J. (2015). *https://www.zliving.com/health/pregnancy-babycare/cow-milk-breast-milk-breast-milk-54477/.*

E., L. (2013). *Digestion Connection.* Rodale.

EATON. (n.d.). *Paleolithic Nutrition. A Consideration of its Nature and Current Implications.* N. Engl. J. Med., 1985312, pp. 283-289.

Goldberg, B. (1998). Chronic Fatigue, Fibromyalgia & Environmental Illness. 101.

Group, E. (2015). *https://globalhealing.com/natural-health/high-fructose-corn-syrup-dangers/#references.*

Gruhier. (2015, November). Ventre fantastique. *Quebec Science*, pp. 20-25.

Gugliucci, A. (2017). *https://academic.oup.com/advances/article/8/1/54/4 566591.*

Guillemette. (2019, october-november). La depression, ce mal insaisissable. *Quebec Science*, pp. 28-33.

Harvey. (2014). *The Connection; Mind your body.* Theconnection.TV.

Heart.org. (2020). *https://www.heart.org/en/healthy-living/healthy-eating/eat-smart/sodium/how-much-sodium-should-i-eat-per-day.*

Hyman. (2013). *Digestion Connection Foreword: Why is your gut making you sick?* Rodale, pp. vii-xi.

Hyman, M. (2009). *The UltaMind Solution.* Scribner, p.177.

Kinnard. (2016, august). Une eau encore bonne à boire? *Quebec Science*, pp. 23-25.

Kleiner, S. (2003). *https://www.menshealth.com/weight-loss/a19518745/weight-loss-high-fructose-corn-syrup/.*

Kresser, C. (2013). *The Paleo Cure.* New York: Little Brown, pp.22.

Kulacz. (2014). *The Toxic Tooth.* MedFox, pp. 155.

Lecavalier, N. L. (n.d.). Giardia and Cryptosporidium in Filtered Drinking Water Supply. *Applied Environmental Microbiology*, 2617-2621.

Letarte. (2019, january). Quand le stress ouvre la porte a la depression. *Quebec Science*, pp. 30-31.

Lipski. (2013). *Digestion Connection.* Rodale, pp. 38.

Martin, J. M. (2000). *Complete Candida Yeast Guidebook.* Three Rivers Press.

Mawer, R. (2019). *https://www.healthline.com/nutrition/why-high-fructose-corn-syrup-is-bad#1.*

MAWER, R. (2019). *https://www.healthline.com/nutrition/why-high-fructose-corn-syrup-is-bad#1.*

Meggs. (2004). *The Inflammation Cure.* McGraw-Hill, pp. 104.

Mesly. (2017, septembre). Glyphosate: la fin d'un règne? *Quebec Science*, pp. 35-39.

Mobbs, A. (2020). *https://www.intelligentlabs.org/fish-oil-dosage/.*

Permutter, D. (2015). *Brain Maker.* New York: Little Brown, p.47, 166.

Rose, J. (1990). *Drinking Water Microbiology.* Sprigner-Verlag.

ROY. (2020, 01). Ce qui cloche avec les implants mammaires. *Protegez-vous*, pp. 18-19.

Seignalet, J. (2012). *L'alimentation ou la troisième médecine.* Éditions Du Rocher, pp. 107, 118, 620.

Seneff. (2019). *GMO's revealed.* [Youtube.com].

Siblerud-Kienholz. (1997). Evidence that Mercury from Silver Dental Fillings may be an Etiological Factor in Reduced Nerve Conduction Velocity in Multiple Sclerosis Patients. *The Journal of Orthomolecular Medicine*, Vol. 12, number 3, p. 169-172.

Smith, J. (2003). *https://pubmed.ncbi.nlm.nih.gov/12870767/.*

Statista. (2018). *https://www.statista.com/statistics/328893/per-capita-consumption-of-high-fructose-corn-syrup-in-the-us/.*

SULLIVAN, D. (2020). *https://www.medicalnewstoday.com/articles/ph-of-blood.*

Teicholz, N. (2014). *https://www.westonaprice.org/health-topics/know-your-fats/the-big-fat-surprise-toxic-heated-oils/.*

themedicalbiochemistrypage.org. (n.d.). *https://themedicalbiochemistrypage.org/minerals-critical-micronutrients/.*

Thompson, C. (2019). *https://www.livestrong.com/article/23346-high-acidic-foods-list/*.

Tremblay, S. (2018, November 19). *http://healthyeating.sfgate.com/healthy-wholewheat-flour-vs-white-3305.html*. Retrieved from http://healthyeating.sfgate.com.

TROTTER, M. C. (2015). *Leaky Gut.* Robert Rose.

Uribarri. (2010, June). Advanced Glycation End Products in Foods and a Practical Guide to their Reduction in the Diet. *American Diet Association*, pp. vol 110: pp. 911-916.

Vasey. (2008). *Gerez votre equilibre acido-basique.* Jouvence, pp. 26.

WANDEL. (2010). *Effects of glucosamine, chondroitin, or placebo in patients with osteoarthritis of hip or knee: network meta-analysis.* BMJ 2010; 341: c4675.

Wright, S. (2019). *https://healthygut.com/articles/how-to-supplement-with-betaine-hcl-for-low-stomach-acid/*.

Yudkin, J. (2012). *Pure, White, and Deadly, p. 38.* Penguin books.

Zelman, K. (2020). *https://www.webmd.com/diet/guide/fiber-how-much-do-you-need#1*.

Printed in Great Britain
by Amazon

31770626R00079